THE MIXED
CRANIAL NERVES

THE MIXED CRANIAL NERVES

Marshall B L Craigmyle MB ChB MD
Formerly Senior lecturer in Anatomy and
Histology, University College, Cardiff,
University of Wales,
and
formerly Visiting Senior Lecturer,
Texas A & M University School of Medicine
College Station, Texas
USA

A Wiley Medical Publication

JOHN WILEY & SONS

Chichester · New York · Brisbane · Toronto · Singapore

British Library Cataloguing in Publication Data:
Craigmyle, Marshall B.L.
  The mixed cranial nerves.
  1.Nerves, cranial
  I.Title
  612'.819   QP381

  ISBN 0 471 90699 9

Library of Congress Cataloging in Publication Data:
Craigmyle, M.B.L. (Marshall Buchanan Lang)
  The mixed cranial nerves.

  (A Wiley medical publication)
  Includes index.
  1. Nerves, Cranial — Anatomy. 2. Nerves, Cranial — Wounds and injuries. I. Title. II.
Series. (DNLM: 1. Cranial Nerves. WL 330 C885m)
  QM571.C73 1985   611'.83   84—29097
  ISBN 0 471 90699 9

CONTENTS

LIST OF ILLUSTRATIONS

PREFACE

In teaching anatomy to medical students and postgraduates for more than thirty years, I have become aware that there are certain spheres of the subject that are regarded as 'difficult'. The difficulty is a conceptual one in the understanding of the tela choroidea or the lesser sac of the peritoneum — in the case of the cranial nerves, the difficulty arises from the complexity of the subject. Over the years, I have evolved a method of presenting the cranial nerves in such a way that my subjects have been able to overcome their difficulty, or so they tell me: this book is a distillation of that method. It covers only the mixed cranial nerves, omitting those cranial nerves concerned with the special senses, and offers a simple and largely pictorial explanation of the permutation of anything from any two from six up to any five from six, which occurs with the mixed cranial nerves.

I am sure that any student who has, perforce, to master the complexities of the mixed cranial nerves will find this book lucid, simple and above all, different in its approach, and he should discover that what is apparently difficult is, in reality, relatively easy. If he does, the book will have justified itself. For each nerve, a section dealing with lesions of that nerve should also help clinical medical students and, perhaps, even their clinical teachers.

M B L CRAIGMYLE
1985

ACKNOWLEDGEMENTS

The germ of this book came from a tape-slide programme of instruction I had prepared whilst on the staff of the Department of Anatomy of University College, Cardiff. I am indebted to Professor J. D. Lever, Chairman and Head of that department for his help, encouragement and constructive criticism. The book would never have come to fruition, however, but for the industry of Mr. Kevin Twohigg, sometime medical illustrator in the above department. The quality of his work which is found throughout the book, speaks for itself. I wish to thank him especially for his tolerance and patience while we worked at the problem of finding the best diagrammatic approach to the subject. I am indebted to Mrs E. Richards and Miss S. Smith for typing the manuscript. I am indebted to Ms. J. Jeffers for typing the index. Finally, to my wife, may I yet again say thanks for her support and encouragement which are as perennial as the grass.

MBLC

1

THE DEVELOPMENT OF THE NERVOUS SYSTEM

The central nervous system is derived from ectoderm. The primordium is a midline antero-posteriorly disposed ectodermal thickening known as the neural plate. The plate sinks into the underlying mesoderm so that it comes to lie in the floor of a groove flanked on either side by raised ridges, the neural folds. The lips of the neural fold bend towards the midline, meet and fuse, the process commencing at the front and extending backwards. In this way a hollow neural tube is formed (Fig 1). The neural tube becomes detached from the overlying ectoderm and so comes to lie free in the underlying mesoderm. As it is doing so, a column of ectodermal cells known as the neural crest forms on either side of the midline in the angle between the neural tube and the ectoderm (Fig 1). The neural crest also becomes detached from the overlying ectoderm and comes to lie free in the mesoderm superolateral to the neural tube on either side. The histogenesis of neural tube and neural crest will now be studied.

HISTOGENESIS OF THE NEURAL TUBE

The neural tube is composed initially of ectodermal cells arranged after a manner reminiscent of a pseudo-stratified columnar epithelium. The tube is covered internally and externally by limiting membranes. At the

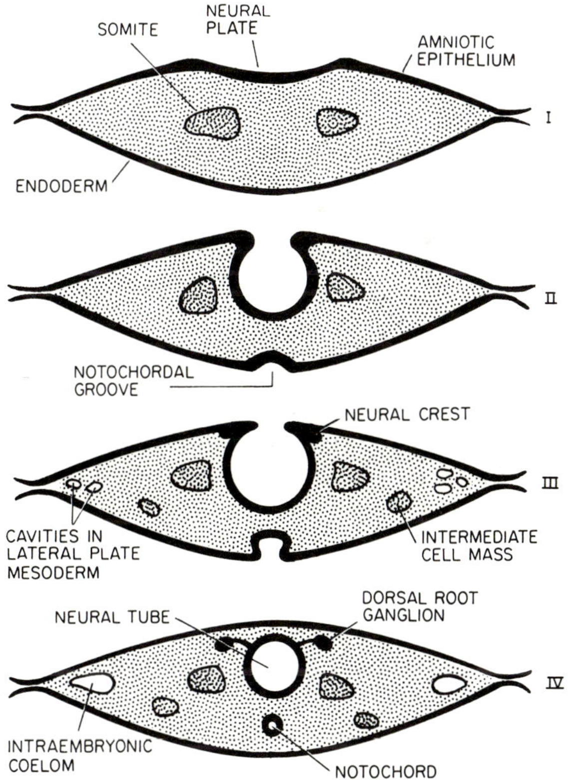

Fig 1 Four stages in the development of the neural tube.

stages of the neural plate and of the very early neural tube, mitotic figures can be seen in the nuclei adjacent to the internal limiting membrane. The mitotic spindles, however, lie in a plane that is paratangential to the internal limiting membrane. The daughter cells resultant upon this division retain contact with one another through terminal bars at the internal limiting membrane. In this way, the neurogenic cells can proliferate, but not differentiate. After the closure of the neural folds, however, the dividing cells near the internal limiting membrane are seen to have a spindle axis which is normal with regard to the plane of the internal limiting membrane. As a result, one of the daughter cells can now lose contact with the other daughter cell and move away from the internal limiting membrane. The daughter cells still in contact with the internal limiting membrane continue to divide in this way, and they constitute the ependymal layer of the developing neural tube. The large numbers of free cells produced in this way constitute the mantle layer of the developing neural tube. These free cells will differentiate into neuroblasts (primitive nerve cells) in the first instance, but will, in later stages of neural tube development, differentiate into spongioblasts (primitive neuroglial cells).

The free neuroblasts initially are rounded and apolar, but later elaborate a juxtaluminal and an abluminal process so that they become bipolar. The abluminal process extends towards the external limiting membrane and is the prospective axon of the cell. It forms, with the corresponding axons from all the other free neuroblasts, an outer fibrous layer to the developing neural tube known as the marginal zone (Fig 2). The neural tube now possesses inner ependymal, middle mantle (future grey matter) and outer marginal (future white matter) layers. The juxtaluminal process of the neuroblast usually regresses so that the cell becomes unipolar. Later the cell body elaborates many small branching processes (dendrites) so that it becomes multipolar.

With the exception of the most cranial section of the developing neural tube, the cells of the mantle zone become disposed in four columns along the length of the tube. Two of these columns are in the dorsolateral aspects of the tube wall which are known as the alar laminae. The other two cell columns lie in the ventrolateral aspects of the tube which are known as the

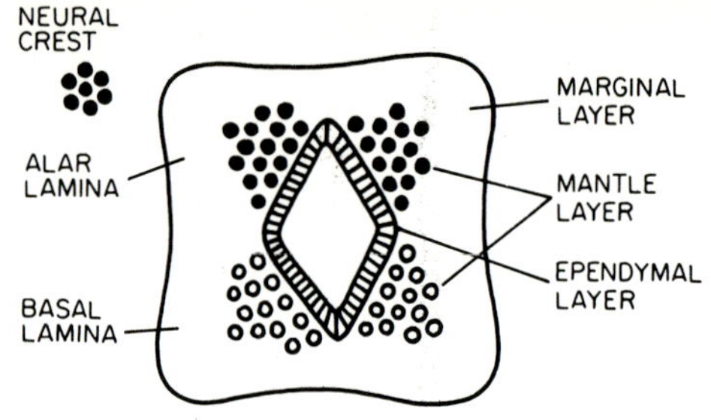

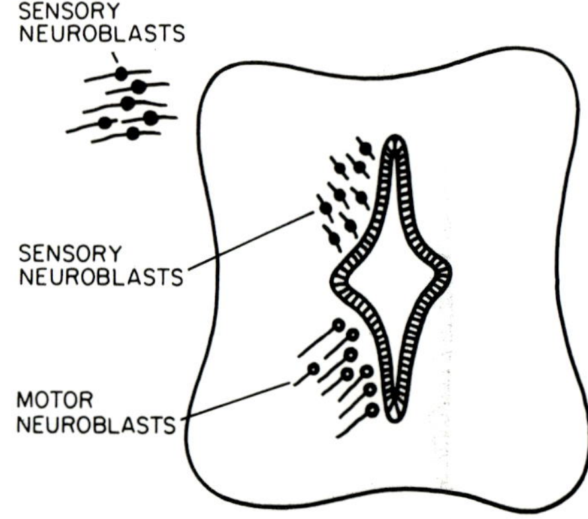

Fig 2   The development of the spinal cord.

basal laminae (Fig 3). The alar lamina on one side is joined to its opposite number by the roof plate, a thin-walled region of the tube where little differentiation has taken place. The basal laminae are joined in similar fashion by a base plate. On each side of the midline, the alar lamina is separated from the basal lamina by an internal groove known as the sulcus limitans (Fig 3).

The axons of the neuroblasts in the basal lamina pass out of the ventrolateral aspect of the tube and enter the adjacent mesenchyme; these constitute the ventral nerve roots. They are destined to terminate in one of two situations:

1   On the myotomic segment of the somite. The myotome will give rise to skeletal muscle fibres and the axons supplying them will be the future lower motor neurones (Fig 3 - D).

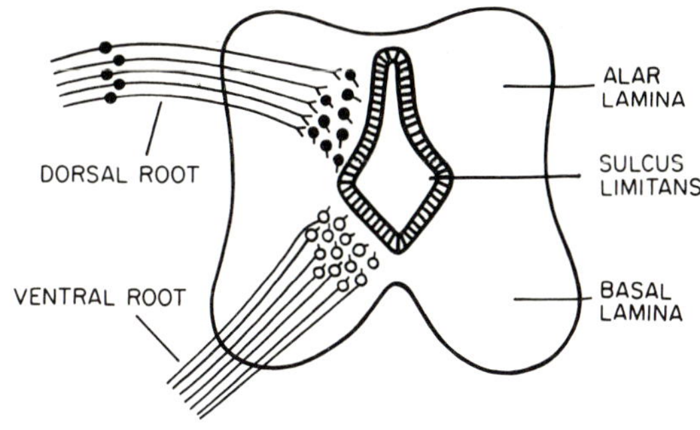

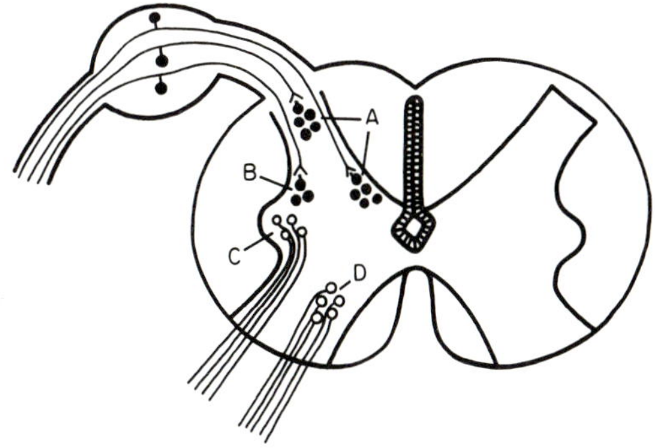

Fig 3   The development of the spinal cord.

2 On those cells of neural crest origin which are destined to become autonomic ganglion cells. In this instance the axons will be the future preganglionic fibres (Fig 3 - C).

The axons of the neuroblasts in the alar lamina, however, tend to remain within the substance of the wall of the neural tube, and to terminate on other neuroblasts within the wall. Those whose axons terminate on neuroblasts at or near the same segmental level as themselves will constitute the intercalated neurones. Those, by contrast, whose axons terminate on neuroblasts at levels higher or lower than themselves will constitute the long ascending and descending sensory tracts.

HISTOGENESIS OF THE NEURAL CREST

The column of cells composing the neural crest becomes aggregated into metameric cell clumps alongside the developing neural tube. Many (but not all) of the neural crest cells will become neuroblasts. They become bipolar in the same way as do the neuroblasts in the wall of the tube, sending one process towards the alar lamina of the developing tube and the other peripherally. The neural crest neuroblast clumps will form the sensory ganglia of the cranial and spinal nerves. The centrally-directed process reaches the alar lamina, penetrates the outer limiting membrane and terminates on a neuroblast in the wall of the neural tube. The distally-directed process grows towards a sensory field in the periphery, and this field may be exteroceptive, interoceptive or proprioceptive. The bipolar neural crest neuroblasts and their processes constitute the dorsal ganglia and roots respectively of the spinal nerve. Later, the neurones of all the sensory ganglia except the vestibulocochlear become pseudo-unipolar by virtue of the merging of the two processes at their origin from the cell body.

2
THE DEVELOPMENT OF THE SPINAL CORD AND BRAIN STEM

SPINAL CORD

This portion of the central nervous system develops from that part of the neural tube caudal to the point where the lips of the neural plate first come together and fuse. At first, neurogenesis within the wall of the tube here is uniform, but it soon becomes localised to the alar and basal laminae. As a result, the tube assumes a rhomboidal appearance (Fig 4). The two alar laminae are in contact with one another by the 30 mm stage: the dorsal portion of the lumen thus becomes obliterated and replaced by the posterior median septum (Fig 4). The basal laminae expand ventrolaterally and are separated by a ventral median sulcus (Fig 4).

By the stage of the 80 mm embryo, the neurones in each basal lamina and in each alar lamina have become subdivided into two longitudinal cell columns as follows:

Alar lamina

(a) A dorsal (general somatic afferent) column which will form the gelatinous substance of Rolando and Clarke's column (Fig 5).

(b) A ventral (general visceral afferent) column (Fig 5).

Basal lamina

(c) A dorsally-placed (general visceral efferent) column which will persist only in the thoracolumbar region and in the sacral region as the lateral horn (Fig 5). The axons of the motor neurones in this column constitute the preganglionic autonomic fibres and leave the spinal cord in the ventral nerve roots.

(d) A ventral (general somatic efferent) column composed of future anterior horn cells (lower motor neurones) whose axons will leave the spinal cord in the ventral roots (Fig 5).

SPINAL NERVES

These are constituted by the amalgamation of the dorsal and ventral roots. The dorsal roots are composed of the centrally-directed (axonic) and the peripherally-directed (dendritic) processes of the pseudo-unipolar nerve cells in the dorsal root ganglion. The fibres conveying interoceptive sensations (from viscera) will constitute the general visceral afferent system. The fibres conveying exteroceptive and proprioceptive sensations will formulate the general somatic afferent system. The ventral

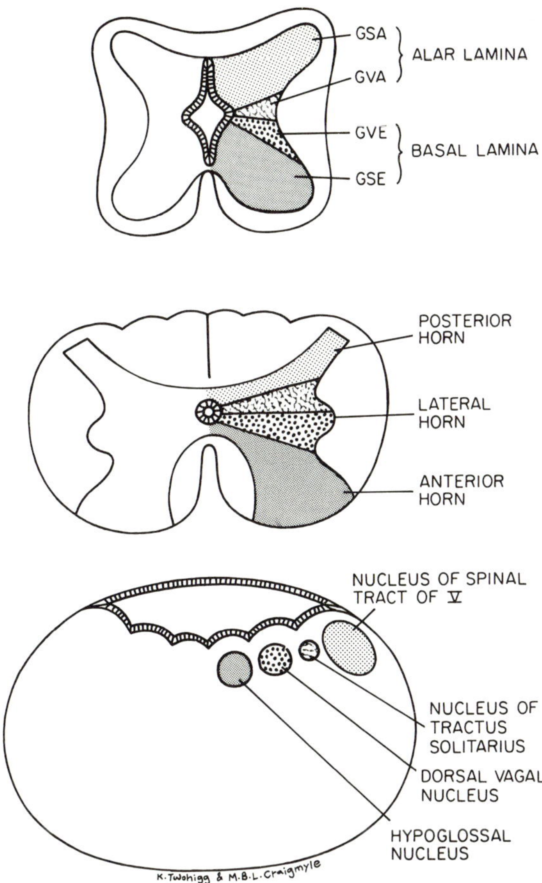

Fig 4   The alar and basal laminae in spinal cord and medulla.

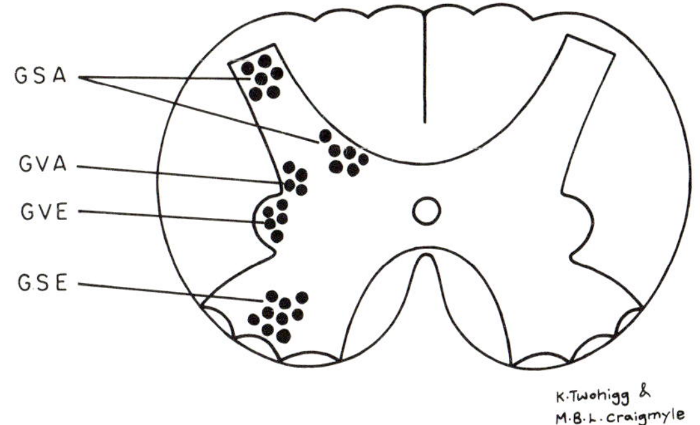

Fig 5   The cell columns in the developing spinal cord.

root is composed of the axons of the general somatic efferent and general visceral efferent groups of nerve cells in the basal lamina.

THE BRAIN STEM

Anterior to the fourth somite, the neural plate shows three bilateral bulgings prior to formation of the neural tube. These become, after closure, the three primary brain vesicles which are, from before backwards, the prosencephalic, mesencephalic and rhombencephalic vesicles. The cranial nerves have their central connections (ie. nuclei) only in the brain stem, that is in those parts of the central nervous system derived from the mesencephalic vesicle (ie. the midbrain) and from the rhombencephalic vesicle (ie. the hindbrain). The rhombencephalon is divisible into a cranial metencephalon from which are developed the cerebellum and pons, and a caudal myelencephalon which will become the medulla oblongata. The cavity of the rhombencephalon will form the fourth ventricle. The floor of the fourth ventricle is formed by the alar and basal laminae of the rhombencephalon, and the nuclei of the fifth to twelfth cranial nerves will lie in the floor of the fourth ventricle. The cavity of the mesencephalon forms the adult cerebral aqueduct. The tectum of the midbrain (future corpora quadrigemina) is formed from the roof plate and alar lamina of the mesencephalon. Alar lamina cells migrate from the metencephalon to the mesencephalon to form the mesencephalic nucleus of the trigeminal nerve. The basal lamina of the mesencephalon will form the nuclei of the third and fourth cranial nerves.

Within the alar and basal laminae of the floor of the brain stem three (not two, as in the spinal cord) longitudinal cell columns develop — ie. there is an extra or special column in each lamina. The additional column in the alar lamina is the special visceral afferent (taste) column. The extra column in the basal lamina is the special visceral (branchial) efferent column. All six columns, represented initially throughout the brain stem, become fragmented into isolated cell clumps which will form the motor and sensory nuclei of the cranial nerves. The brain stem representation of the six columns is presented in Fig 6.

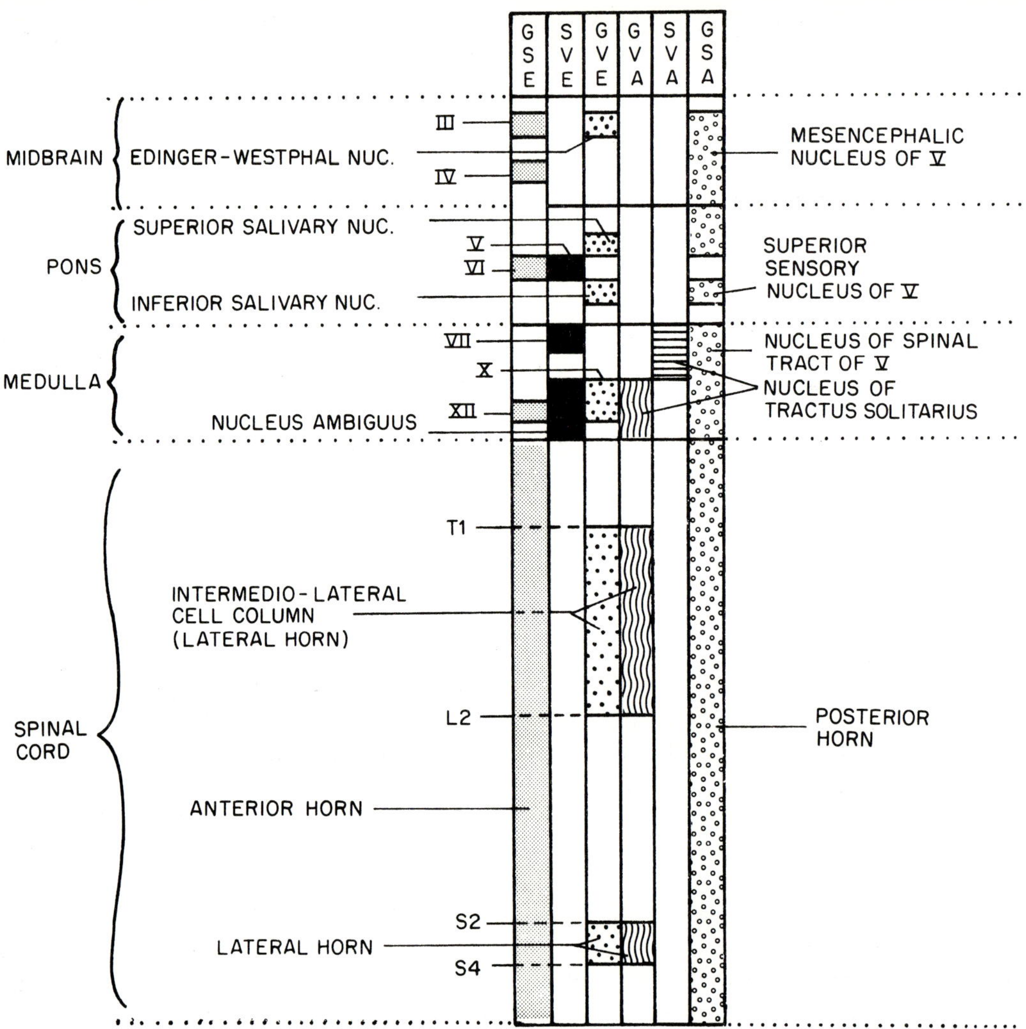

Fig 6   The general and special columns in the brain stem and spinal cord.

3
THE CELL COLUMNS OF THE SPINAL CORD

Four longitudinal cell columns form in the developing spinal cord, two in the *alar* lamina (ie. general somatic afferent and general visceral afferent) and two in the *basal* lamina (ie. general somatic efferent and general visceral efferent). Of these columns, the two somatic columns occur throughout the length of the spinal cord in the adult, but the general visceral efferent and general visceral afferent columns persist in only two situations:

(a) As the lateral horn (intermedio-lateral cell column) between cord segments T1 and L2 inclusive. The motor nerve cells here give rise to *sympathetic* preganglionic fibres.

(b) As the lateral horn at spinal cord segments S2 and S3. The motor nerve cells here give rise to *parasympathetic* preganglionic fibres.

BASIC PATTERN OF VISCEROCEPTIVE, EXTEROCEPTIVE AND PROPRIOCEPTIVE SENSATIONS

The sensory pathway between the periphery and the cerebral cortex is constituted by three neurones in series and called first, second and third-order in succession, so that two synapses are involved. The cell bodies of the three neurones are to be found:

First Order Neurone:

In the ganglion of the dorsal root of the spinal nerve (Fig 7).

Second Order Neurone:

In the posterior grey column of the spinal cord or in the cranial extension of this column in the medulla oblongata and pons (Fig 7).

Third Order Neurone:

In the contralateral thalamus (Fig 7).

Thus, while the cell body of the first order neurone lies in the peripheral nervous system, the cell bodies of the second and third order neurones are located in the central nervous system and, therefore, both synapses lie within the central nervous system. The first order neurone is pseudounipolar and its central process enters the central nervous system before relaying. The site of the first synapse depends on the type of sensation being carried:

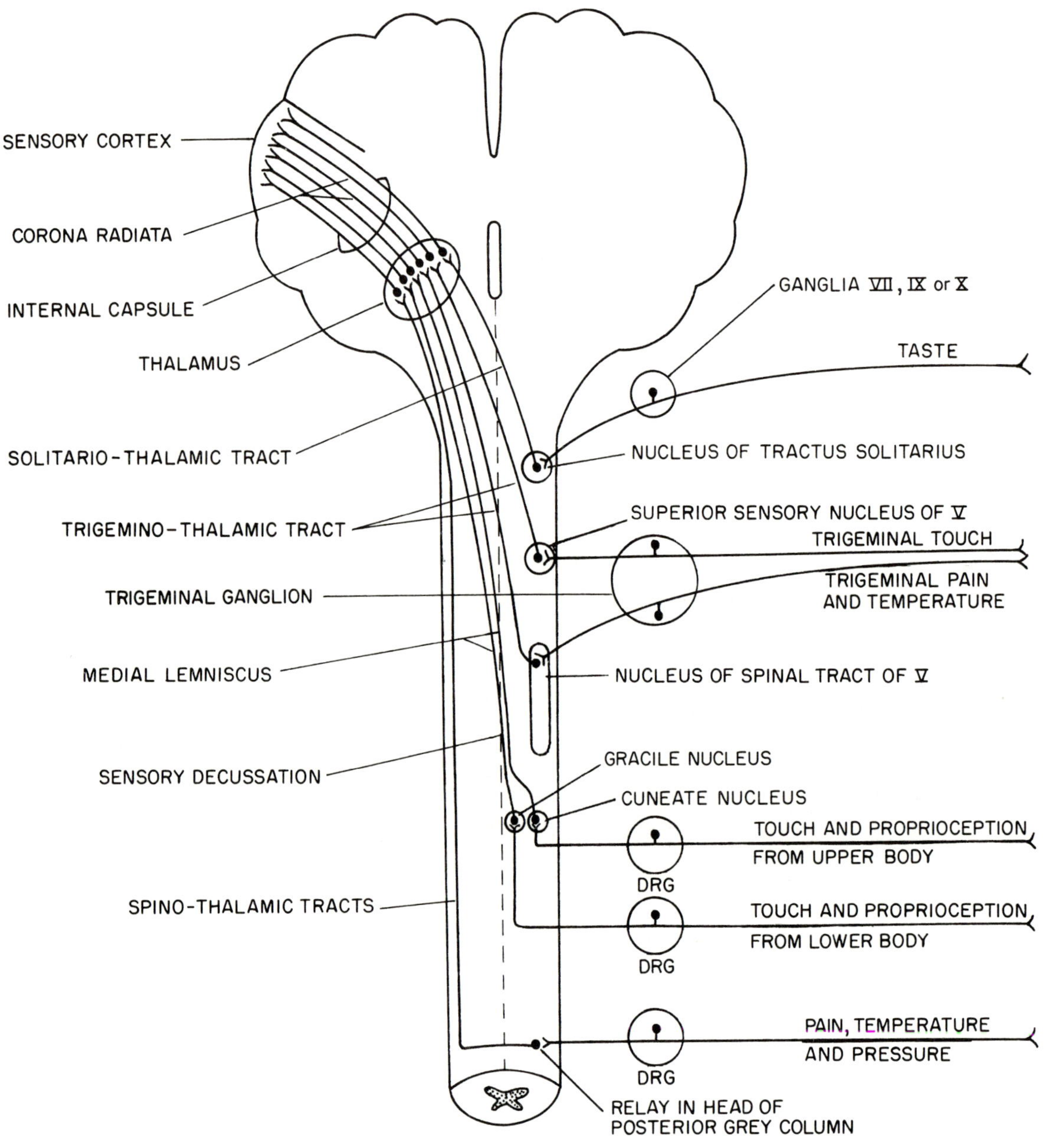

Fig 7   The three-neurone chain of the sensory pathways.

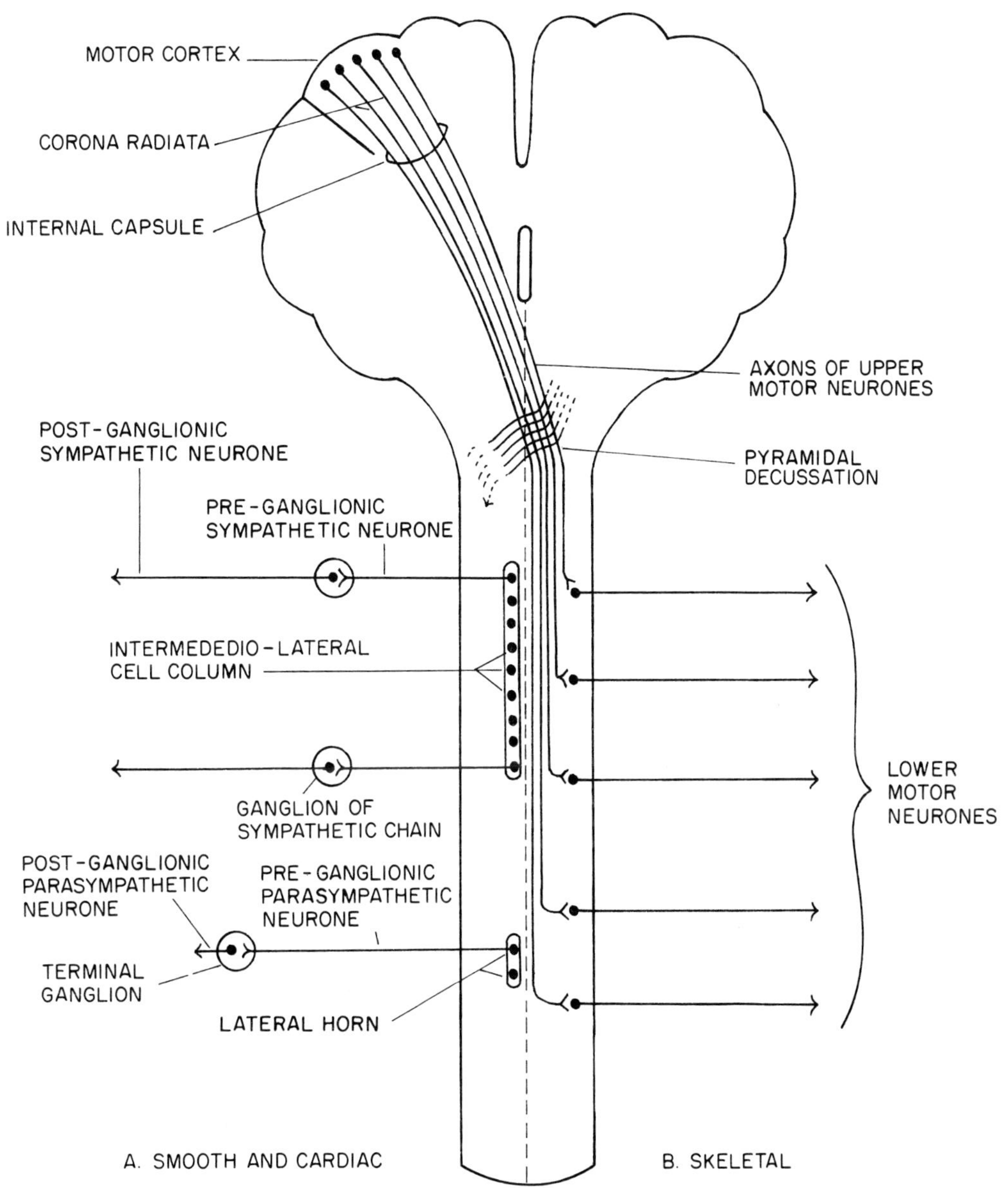

Fig 8 The two-neurone chain of the motor pathways.

The general somatic afferent column (exteroceptive and proprioceptive impulses)

The first synapse is to be found for:

(a) temperature — posterior horn of spinal cord,
(b) pain — posterior horn of spinal cord,
(c) touch — gracile and cuneate nuclei of the medulla, and
(d) proprioception — in the gracile and cuneate nuclei of the medulla.

The general visceral afferent column (interoceptive impulses)

The first synapse is to be found at the base of the posterior horn of the spinal cord.

BASIC PATTERN OF SPINAL NERVE MOTOR PATHWAYS

Voluntary muscle (Fig 8 - A)

Skeletal muscle derived from somites is innervated by the general somatic efferent pathway, is composed of two neurones in series, with a synapse between. These are known as the upper and lower motor neurones. The cell body of the upper motor neurone lies in layer 5 of the motor cortex, which occupies the precentral gyrus of the cerebral cortex. Its axon passes, via the corona radiata and the internal capsule, into the basis pedunculi of the cerebral peduncle. From there it passes down through the pons, and in the medulla oblongata crosses the midline, decussating with its opposites in the pyramidal decussation. Thereafter the upper motor neurone axons form the pyramidal tract of the opposite side of the spinal cord, and terminate by synapsing on the cell bodies of the anterior horn. These cells comprise the lower motor neurones. Their axons pass out of the spinal cord in the ventral roots of the spinal nerves and terminate on the motor end-plate of anything between 1 and 100 skeletal muscle fibres. The ratio of axon to muscle fibre is 1:1 in the case of such muscles as the lumbricals where fine movement is the norm and may go as high as 1:100 (ie. the axon branches into 100 terminals each of which goes to a different skeletal muscle fibre) in muscles like gluteus maximus where gross movements occur.

Involuntary muscle (Fig 8 - B)

Smooth and cardiac muscle fibres are also innervated by two neurones in series. Because, however, the cell body of the first order neurone lies in the central nervous system whereas the cell body of the second order neurone lies in a ganglion of the peripheral nervous system, the two neurones are designated as preganglionic and postganglionic respectively. The origin of the preganglionic fibres of the autonomic nervous system from within the spinal cord is not from a single continuous column but is the outflow from two separate masses, viz:

1   The lateral horn (intermediolateral cell column) between the first thoracic and second lumbar segments of the spinal cord.
2   The lateral horn which lies opposite the second, third and fourth sacral segments of the spinal cord.

The general somatic efferent column (*innervation of skeletal muscle,* Fig 8 - B)

The general somatic efferent column is composed of the single continuum of anterior horn cells, or lower motor neurones. Their axons leave the spinal cord in the ventral roots and pass along the mixed peripheral nerves to terminate on the motor end plate of up to 100 skeletal muscle fibres.

The general visceral efferent column (*innervation of smooth and cardiac muscle,* Fig 8 - A)

The general visceral efferent column consists of the intermediolateral cell column between spinal cord segments T1—L2 inclusive, the cells of which give rise to preganglionic *sympathetic* fibres. The second representation of the column is the lateral horn at S2 and 3, which gives rise to *parasympathetic* preganglionic fibres. Both sets of fibres synapse on ganglion cells in the peripheral nervous system after leaving the spinal cord in the ventral root. In general, the sympathetic preganglionic axon is short and the postganglionic axon is long: in other words, the sympathetic ganglia lie close to the central nervous system. They lie in the sympathetic chain (paravertebral ganglia) and close to the abdominal aorta (collateral ganglia such as the coeliac, mesenteric and renal). In contrast, the parasympathetic preganglionic fibre is long and the postganglionic fibre short: so short, indeed, that the ganglia of origin of the postganglionic fibres lie most commonly in the wall of the viscus being supplied (terminal ganglia).

Mixed peripheral nerves entering the limbs contain postganglionic sympathetic fibres but *are devoid of parasympathetic fibres.* The sympathetic fibres in any mixed limb nerve can be classified as being of three types:

Vasomotor: these supply the smooth muscle of the blood vessels of the limb and are vasoconstrictor in function.

Pilomotor: these supply the smooth (arrectores pilorum) muscles of the skin of the limb.

Sudomotor: these supply the myoepithelial cells of the sweat glands in the limb.

Sympathetic fibres from the outflow between T1 and L2 provide the sympathetic supply to the entire body.

Parasympathetic fibres from the outflow between S2 and S4 give rise to the pelvic splanchnic nerves (or nervi erigentes). These provide the parasympathetic nerve supply to that part of the alimentary canal derived from the hindgut (ie. splenic flexure, descending colon, sigmoid colon and rectum) and to the pelvic viscera. (The tenth cranial nerve, or vagus nerve, supplies the parasympathetic fibres to foregut, midgut and all other abdominal and all thoracic viscera.)

4
THE GENERAL CELL COLUMNS IN THE BRAIN STEM

The general somatic afferent column (Fig 9)

This, the posterior grey column of the spinal cord, extends into the medulla oblongata as the nucleus of the spinal tract of the trigeminal nerve, as the nucleus gracilis and the nucleus cuneatus. The last two nuclei do not extend into the pons, unlike the nucleus of the spinal tract of the trigeminal nerve. It becomes slender as it ascends and terminates at mid-pons by expanding to form the main sensory nucleus of the trigeminal nerve (Fig 10).

As one moves from neck to head, the somatic sensory function of the second cervical nerve (C1 has no cutaneous representation) is succeeded by the trigeminal nerve. The dorsal root ganglion of C2 is in series with the trigeminal ganglion. Both contain pseudounipolar nerve cells. There is one significant difference, however, in that whereas the cell body of the first order neurone on the **proprioceptive** pathway of C2 lies in the dorsal root ganglion of that nerve, the cell body of the first order neurone on the *trigeminal* **proprioceptive** pathway lies in the mesencephalic nucleus of the trigeminal nerve. This is a long slender column of pseudounipolar cells which extends from the superior sensory nucleus of the trigeminal nerve at the level of the middle pons, up to the mid-brain lateral to the aqueduct (Fig 10).

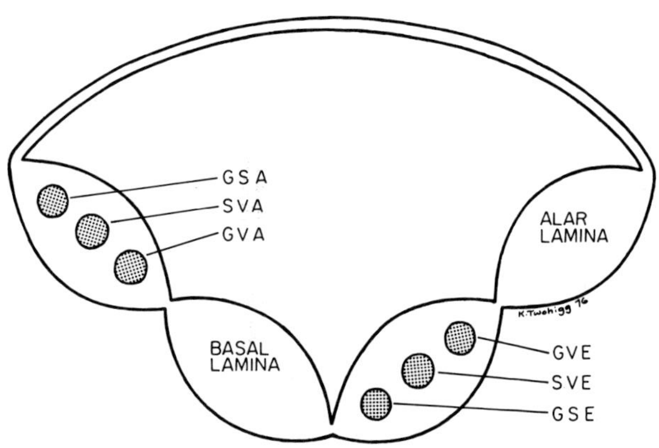

Fig 9 The general and special columns in the brain stem.

The general visceral afferent column (Fig 9)

This is represented in the brain stem by a slender column in the medulla, the nucleus of the tractus solitarius (Fig 11). The fibres which end in the *lower* part of this nucleus are the central processes of the pseudo-unipolar nerve cells in the inferior ganglion of the glosso-pharyngeal nerve and the inferior ganglion of the vagus nerve (ganglion nodosum). They convey sensations, other than taste, from all the viscera but principally of

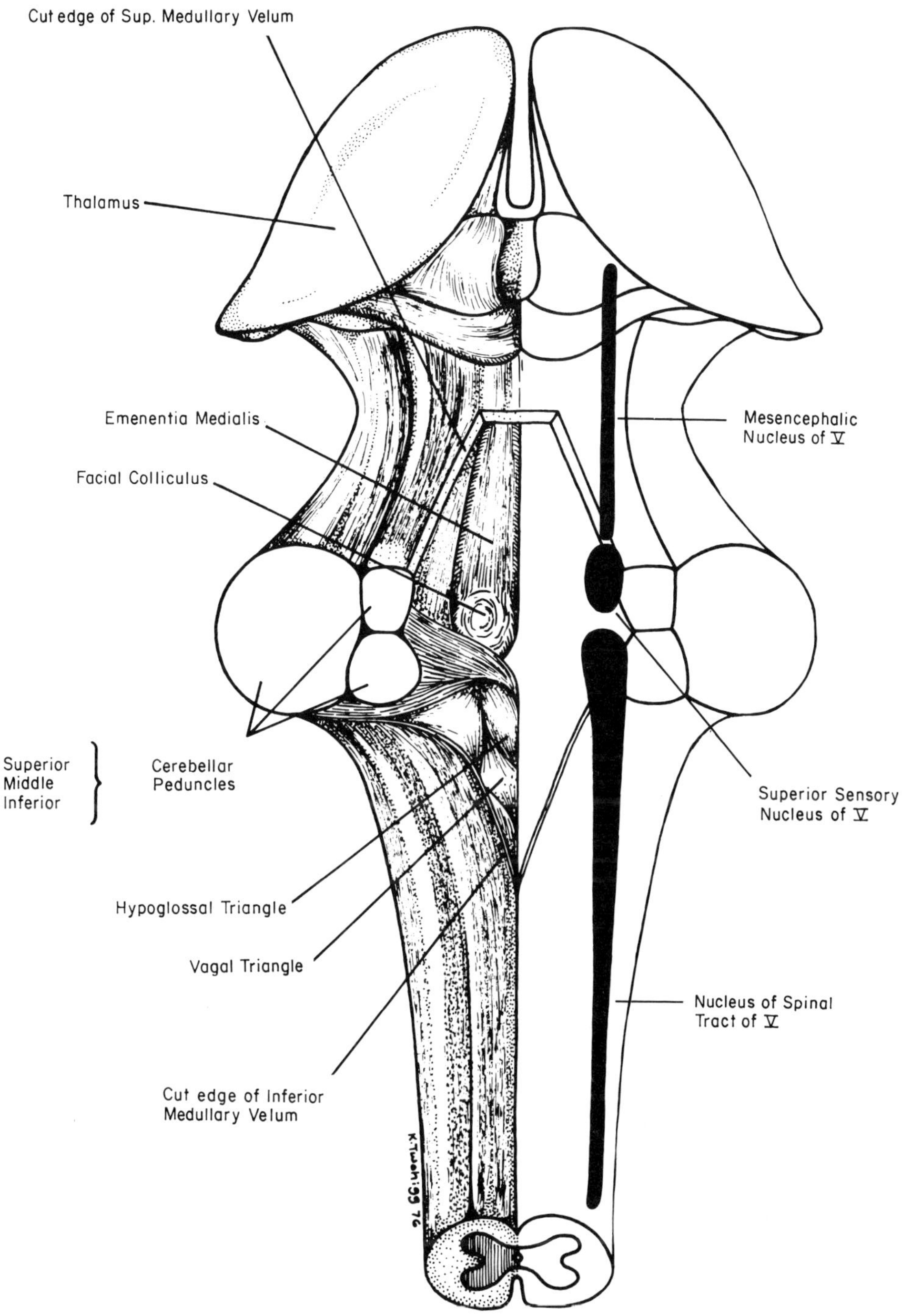

Fig 10   The general somatic afferent column in the brain stem.

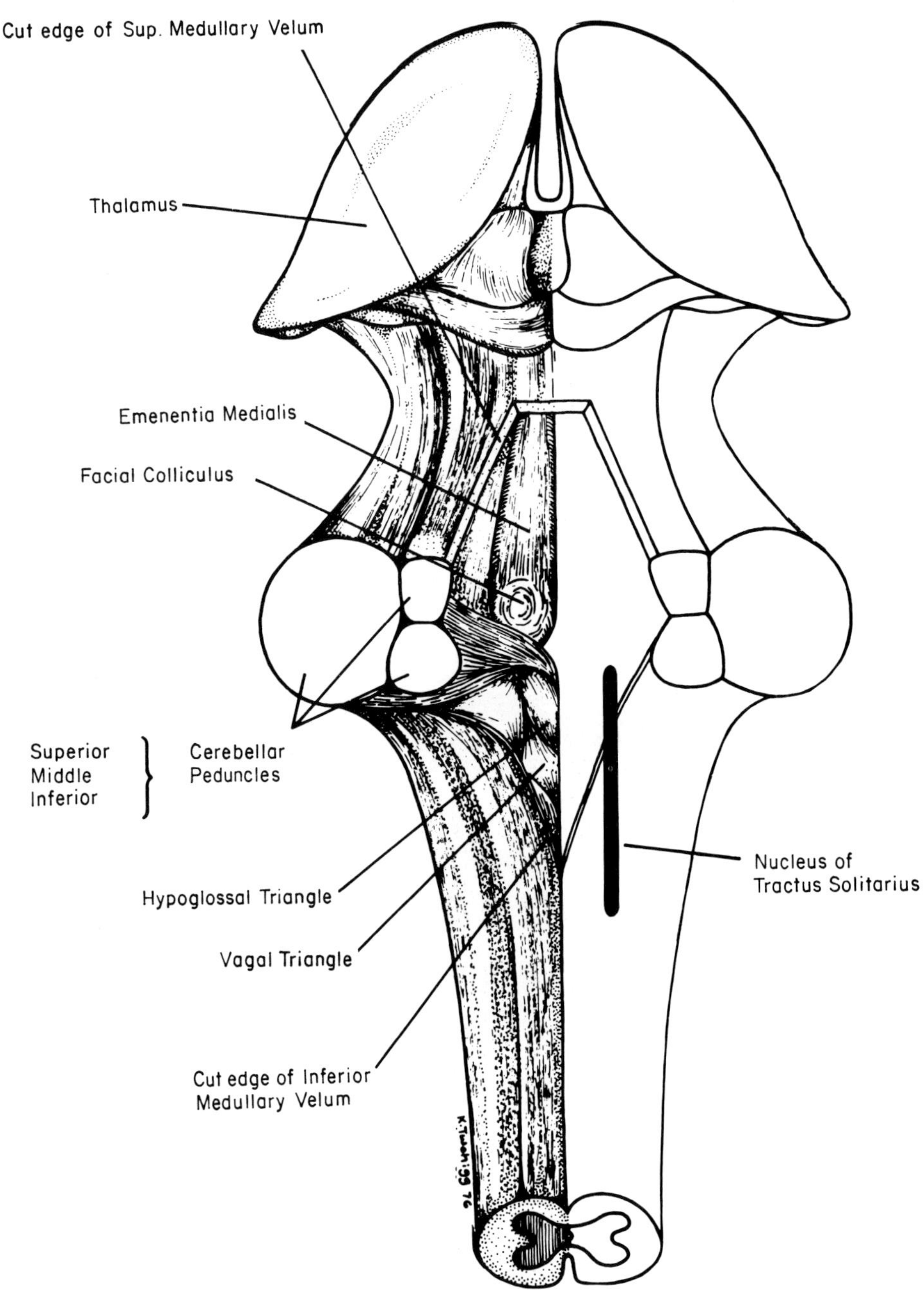

Fig 11   The general visceral afferent column in the brain stem.

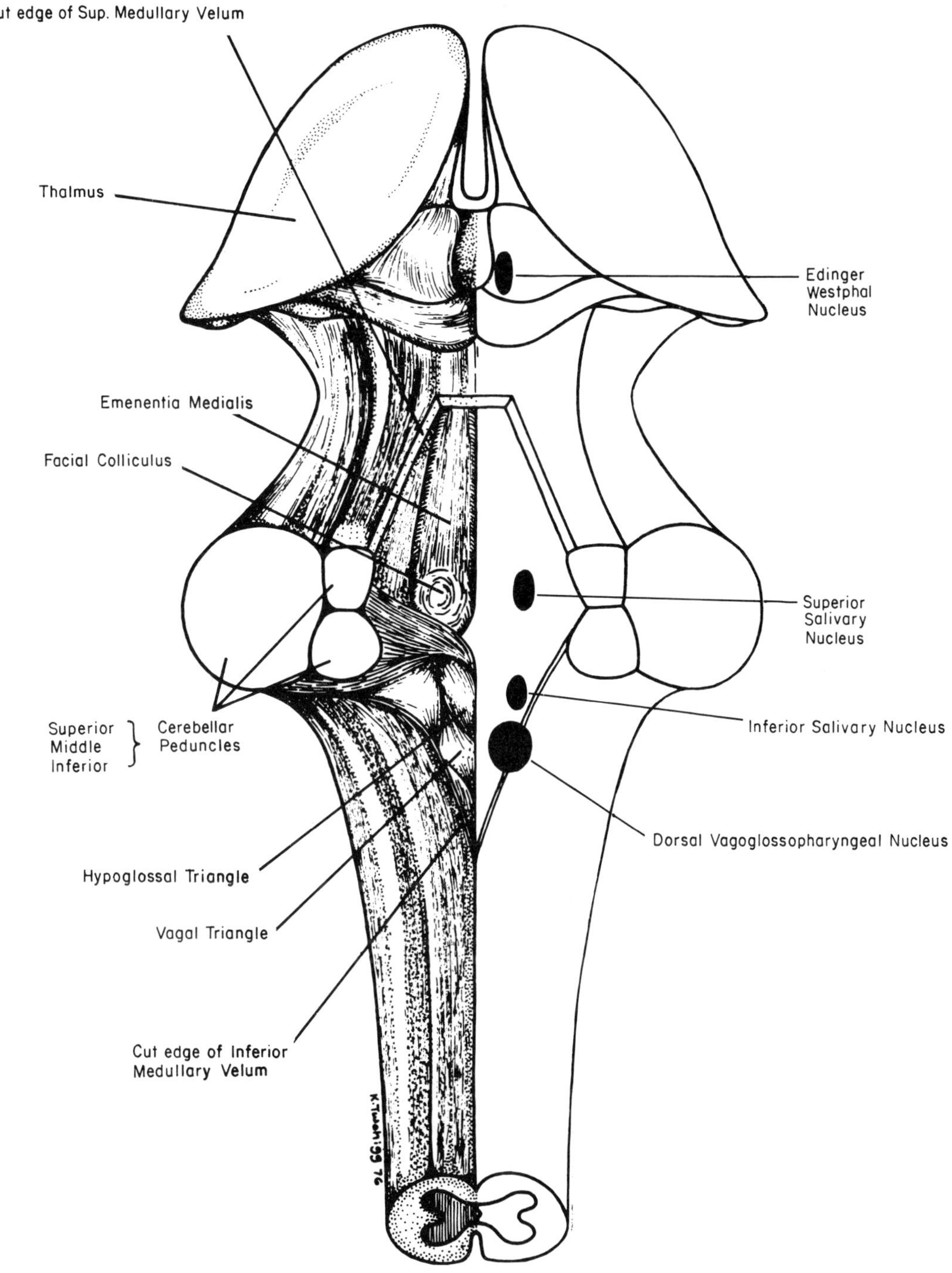

Fig 12 The general visceral efferent column in the brain stem.

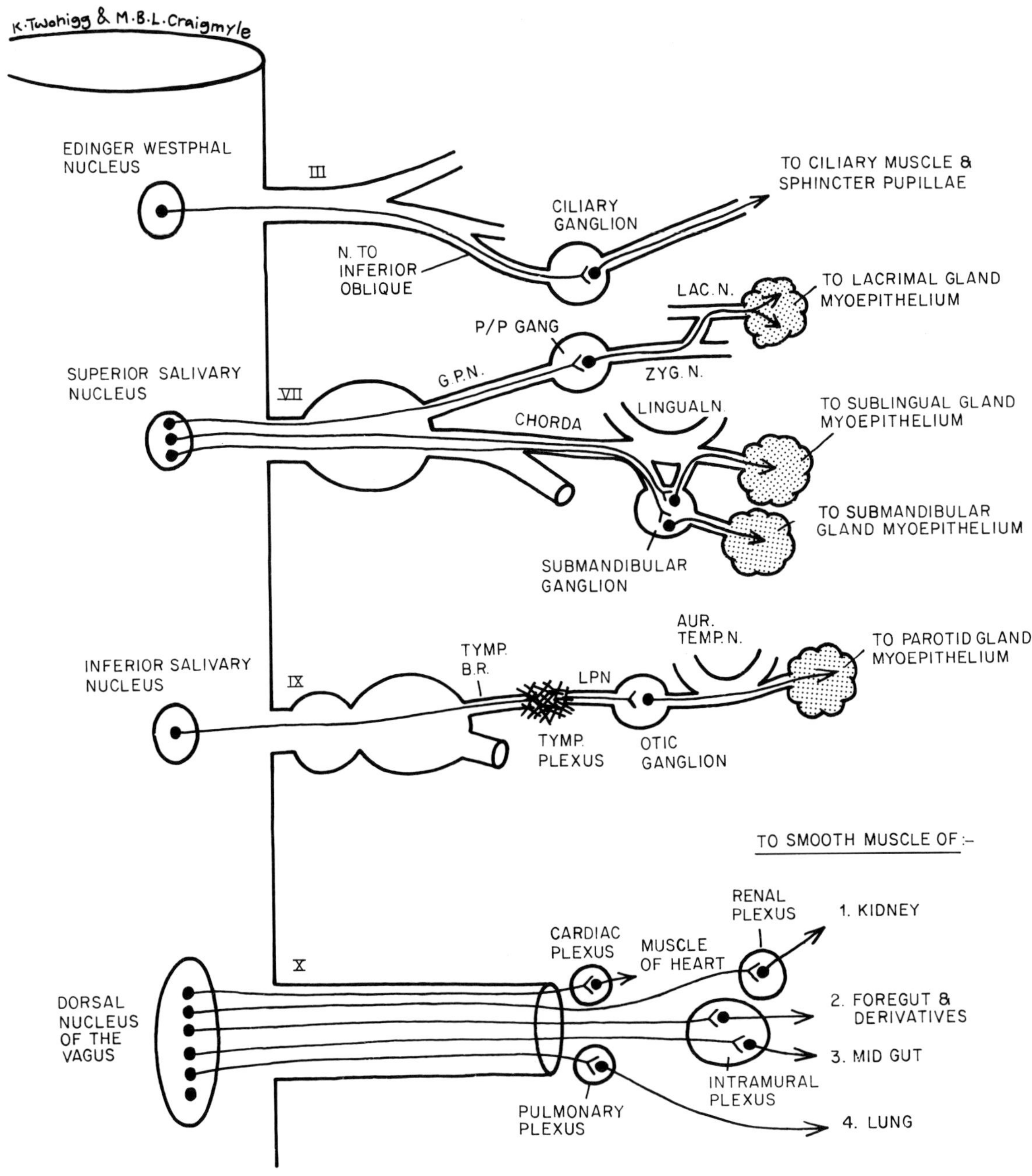

Fig 13   The general visceral efferent pathways from the brain stem.

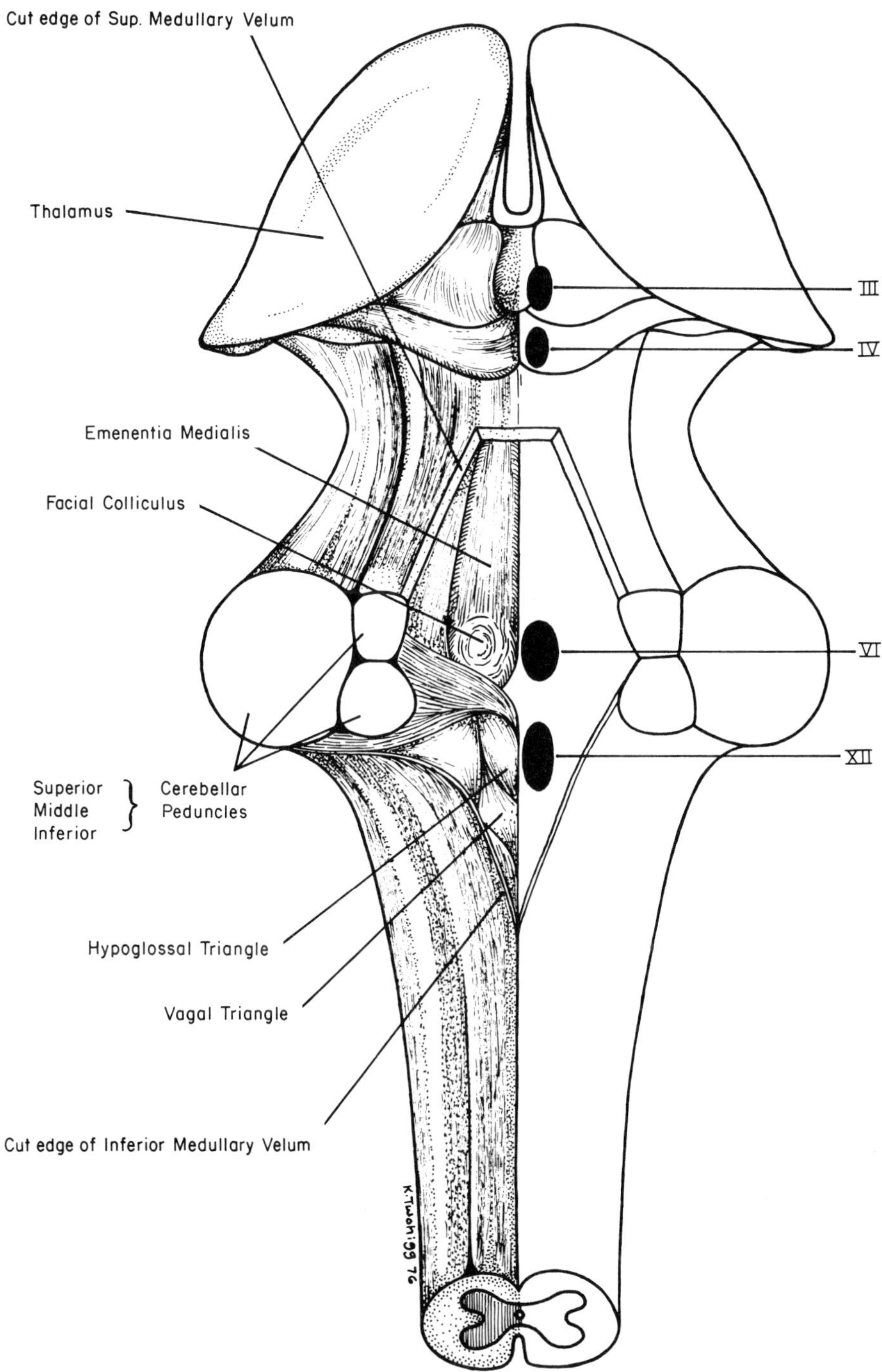

Fig 14 The general somatic efferent column in the brain stem.

course that will mean from the alimentary canal and respiratory tract and their upper expanded portions, ie. mouth, nose and pharynx.

The general visceral efferent column (Fig 9)

This column, which is motor to involuntary muscle and is represented in the spinal cord by the lateral horn from T1—L2 and from S2 to S4, is present in the brain stem as four discrete nuclei which from below upwards, are (Fig 12):

> the dorsal motor nucleus of the vagus
> the inferior salivary nucleus
> the superior salivary nucleus
> the Edinger-Westphal nucleus

All four nuclei give rise to preganglionic parasympathetic fibres, as does the lateral horn at S2—4 and the five nuclei taken as a group constitute the *craniosacral* (parasympathetic) outflow of the autonomic nervous system (the fibres from T1—L2 represent the (sympathetic) *thoracolumbar* outflow of the autonomic nervous system). The position of, and distribution of the fibres from, the four brain-stem nuclei is as follows:

(a)   Dorsal motor nucleus of the vagus

This nucleus lies in the medullary part of the floor of the fourth ventricle, its upper part causing a small impression on the floor of the ventricle, the vagal triangle. The preganglionic axons from the cells in the nucleus leave the brain stem in the vagal and cranial accessory nerves, which join. They are distributed to the striped muscle of the heart, and to the smooth muscle of thoracic viscera, abdominal viscera and those portions of the alimentary canal derived from foregut and midgut. The fibres synapse with nerve cells located in the cardiac ganglia or in the walls of the viscera concerned (terminal ganglia). These nerve cells give rise to short postganglionic fibres which supply the cardiac muscle or the viscus, as applicable (Fig 13).

(b)   The inferior salivary nucleus

This small collection of nerve cells lies in the medulla,

dorsolateral to the hypoglossal nucleus. Its preganglionic parasympathetic fibres pass to the glossopharyngeal nerve, reach the otic ganglion in its lesser petrosal branch, and relay there. The postganglionic fibres are secretomotor to the parotid gland (Fig 13).

(c)   The superior salivary nucleus

This is also a small nucleus, located in the pons dorsolateral to the facial nucleus. Its axons pass to the facial nerve and relay either in the pterygopalatine or the submandibular ganglion. Postganglionic fibres pass from these ganglia to the lacrimal gland and the submandibular and sublingual salivary glands (Fig 13). The salivary glands of the nose and palate are also supplied by postganglionic fibres from the pterygopalatine ganglion, but these in the interests of simplification, have not been shown in the diagram.

(d)   The Edinger-Westphal nucleus

This small nucleus is comma-shaped and lies medial to the upper end of the oculomotor nucleus. Its axons pass into the oculomotor nerve, relay in the episcleral or ciliary ganglion and the postganglionic fibres supply the smooth muscle of the ciliary body and sphincter pupillae (Fig 13).

The general somatic efferent column (Fig 9)

This column of lower motor neurones which exists to supply skeletal muscle derived from somites, and which is analagous with the anterior horn cells of the spinal cord, is found as four nuclei in the brain stem. These are, from below upwards (Fig 14):

> the hypoglossal nucleus — in the upper medulla
> the abducent nucleus — in the lower pons
> the trochlear nucleus — in the lower midbrain
> the oculomotor nucleus — in the upper midbrain

The hypoglossal nucleus supplies all the intrinsic and all the extrinsic tongue muscles except palatoglossus. The abducent, trochlear and oculomotor nuclei collectively supply all the extrinsic ocular muscles and the oculomotor nerve also supplies the levator palpebrae superioris. All these muscles, including those of the tongue, are derived from the occipital somites.

5

THE SPECIAL COLUMNS IN THE BRAIN STEM

The special visceral afferent column (Fig 15)

This column, which is not represented in the spinal cord, exists to subserve the function of taste (*and proprioception from the skeletal muscles derived from branchial arch mesoderm: since, however, the fibres in the latter group are usually described under the general somatic afferent heading, this convention will be followed here*). The column is composed of the *upper* part of the nucleus of the tractus solitarius, a long column of cells in the medulla (Fig 16). The fibres reaching the nucleus are the central processes of pseudo-unipolar nerve cells located in the inferior ganglion of the vagus nerve, the inferior ganglion of the glossopharyngeal nerve and the facial (geniculate) ganglion. The vagus carries taste fibres from the epiglottis. The glossopharyngeal nerve subserves taste from the posterior one-third of the tongue. The facial nerve carries taste from the presulcal tongue and from the palate: the fibres enter the brain stem in the sensory root (nervus intermedius) of the nerve en route for the nucleus of the tractus solitarius.

The special visceral (branchial) efferent column (Fig 17)

This column of lower motor neurones exists to supply skeletal muscle derived from *branchial arch* mesoderm. It is found as three nuclei in the brain stem which, from above downwards, are (Fig 18):

> the *motor nucleus of the trigeminal nerve* — in the mid-pons
> the *facial nucleus* — in the lower pons
> the *nucleus ambiguus* — in the medulla

The motor nucleus of the trigeminal nerve sends its axons to the mandibular division of the trigeminal nerve, which is the nerve of the first branchial arch, and supplies the muscles of mastication and the other first arch muscles (tensor tympani; tensor palati; mylohyoid; anterior belly of digastric) (Fig 18). The facial nerve is the nerve of the second branchial arch. It supplies the second arch muscles: muscles of facial expression; buccinator; stapedius; stylohyoid; posterior belly of digastric. The nucleus ambiguus represents the fused nuclei of the hinder branchial arches: it sends fibres to the third arch nerve (glossopharyngeal) for the innervation of stylopharyngeus and to the accessory (nerve of fourth arch) and vagus (nerve of sixth arch) for the supply of the skeletal muscle of the palate, pharynx, larynx, and oesophagus (Fig 18), as well as the sternomastoid and trapezius muscles in all probability.

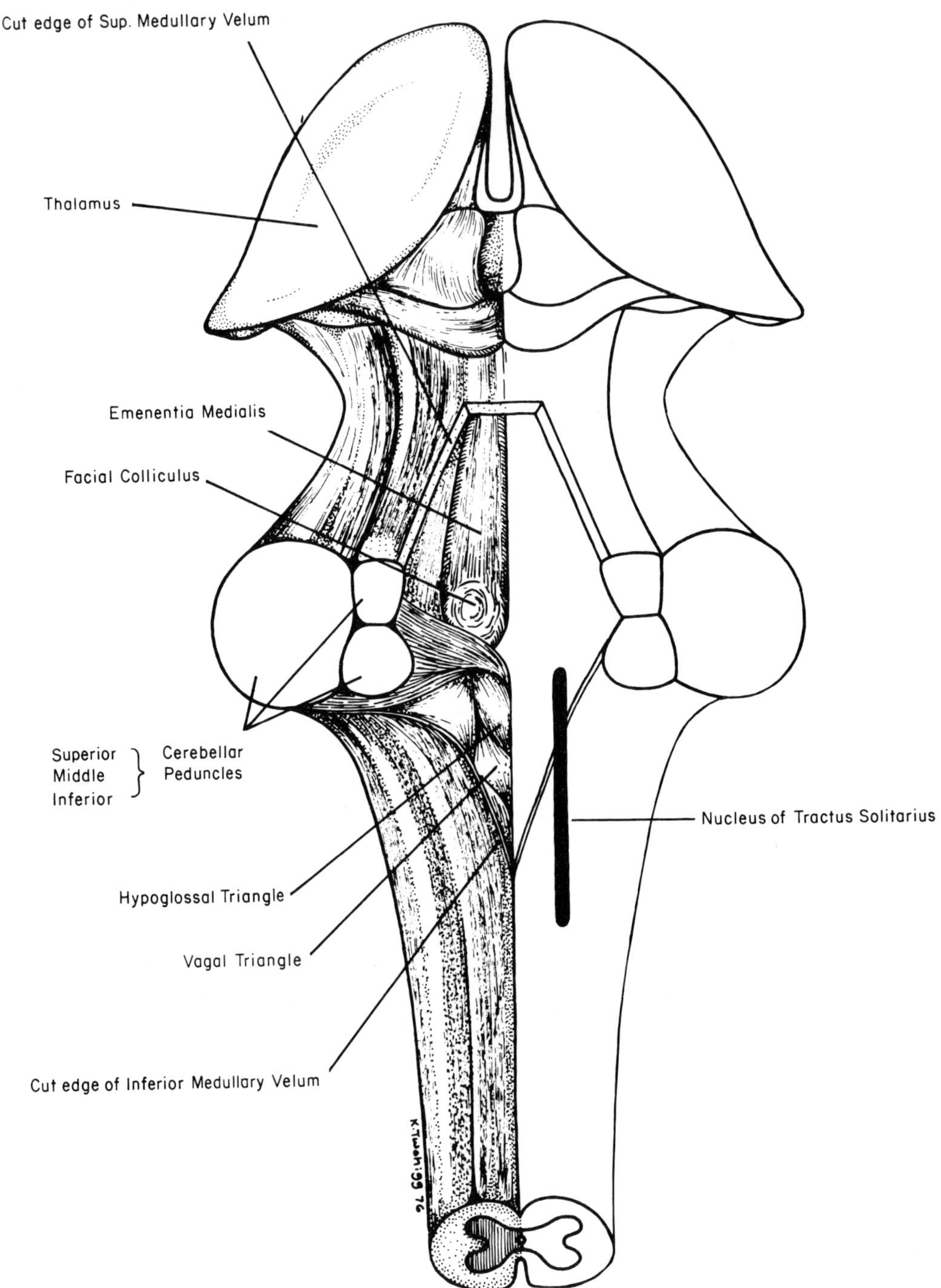

Fig 15   The special visceral afferent (taste) column in the brain stem.

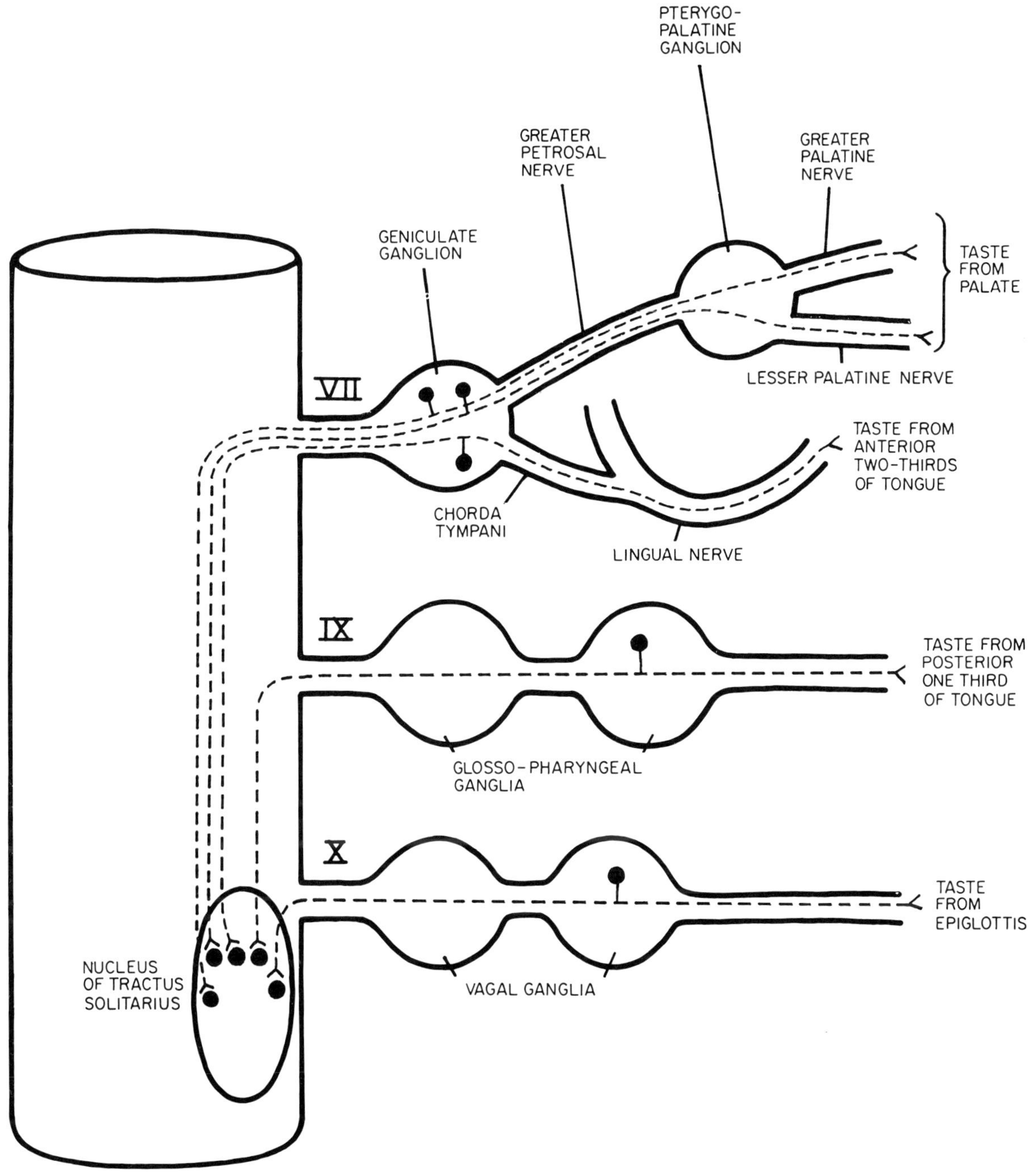

Fig 16   The special visceral afferent (taste) pathways.

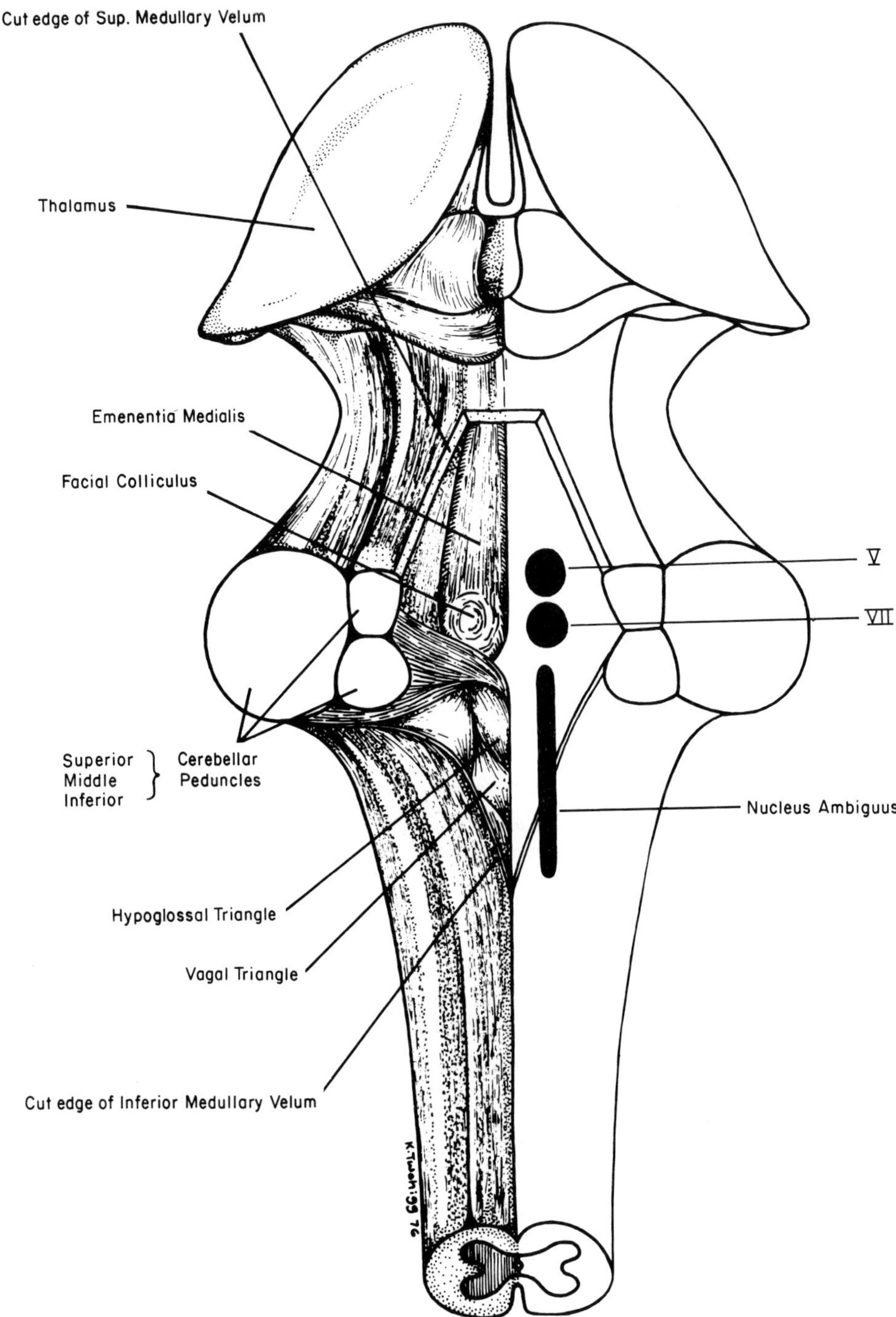

Fig 17   The special visceral (branchial) efferent column in the brain stem.

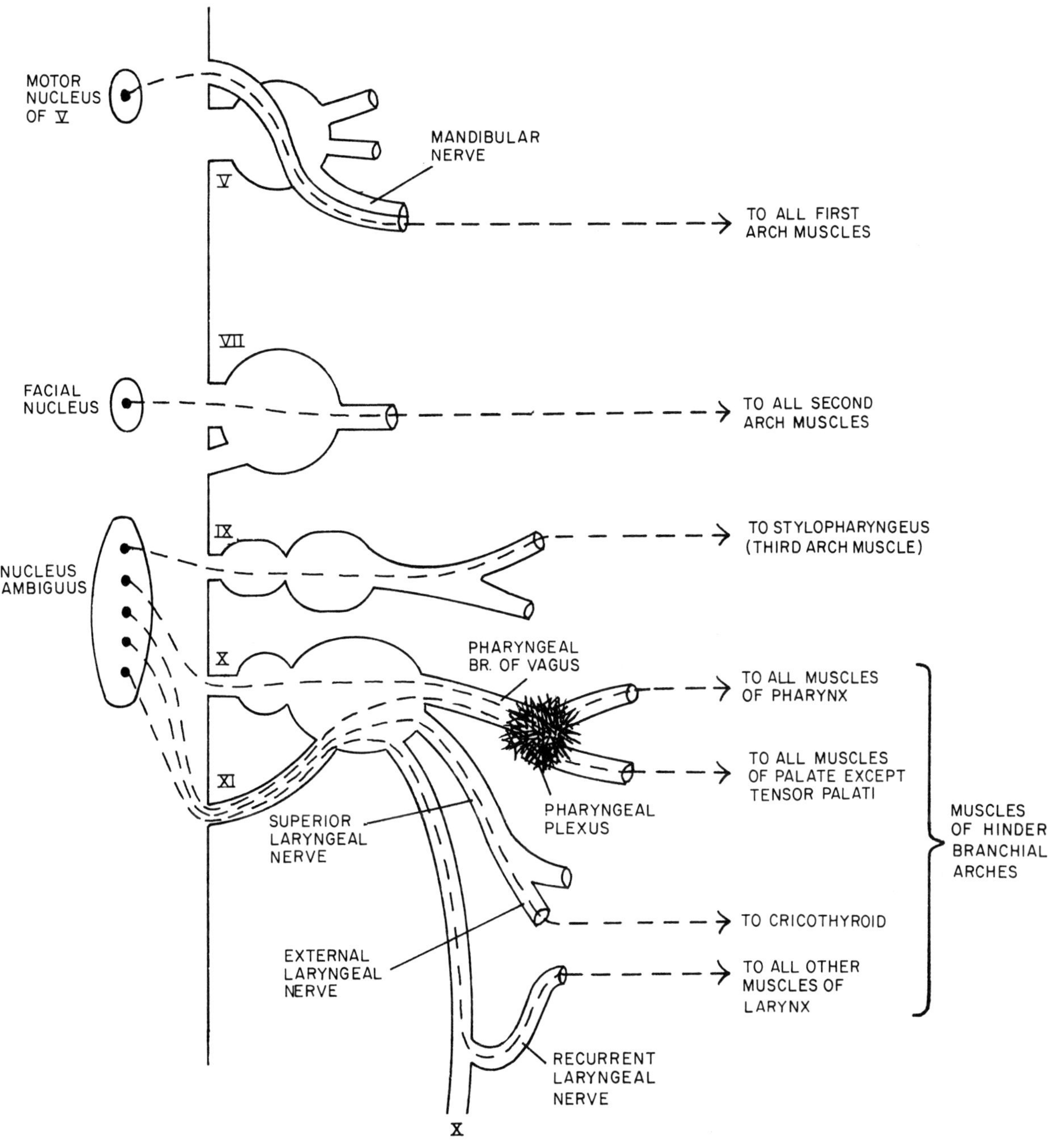

Fig 18   The special visceral (branchial) efferent pathways.

6

THE DEEP CONNECTIONS OF THE CRANIAL NERVES

The various nuclei derived from persistent sections of the general and special columns of the brain stem and spinal cord comprise the nuclear connections of the cranial nerves. All these nuclei have complex deeper connections and also connections with the nuclei of other cranial nerves. No attempt has been made in the ensuing chapters, which deal with the cranial nerves individually, to enumerate the deeper connections of each cranial nerve: this has been done in the interests of simplicity. Certain basic rules can however be applied to all the mixed cranial nerves.

MOTOR NUCLEI

1 All motor nuclei receive afferents from the motor cortex of the same side via the corticonuclear tract if the nucleus lies in the brain stem, and via the corticospinal tract if the nucleus lies in the spinal cord.
2 All motor nuclei have connections with the extrapyramidal system.
3 All motor nuclei have connections with other motor nuclei concerned with the same function.
4 All motor nuclei have connections with sensory nuclei concerned with the same function or region.
5 All cranial nerves containing parasympathetic efferent fibres will have connections with the hypothalamus.

SENSORY NUCLEI

1 All sensory nuclei are connected to the sensory cortex via the thalamus.
2 All sensory nuclei have connections with the reticular formation.
3 All sensory nuclei are connected to motor nuclei serving the same region or function.
4 All sensory nerves containing proprioceptive fibres are connected with the cerebellum.
5 All sensory nuclei are connected to the hypothalamus if they are visceroceptive nuclei.

7

THE OCULOMOTOR NERVE

ORIGIN, COURSE AND DISTRIBUTION

The oculomotor nerve arises from the midbrain from the medial side of the basis pedunculi (Fig 19) as a series of rootlets. The nerve passes into the interpeduncular cistern of the subarachnoid space. After passing between the posterior cerebral and superior cerebellar arteries, the nerve pierces the arachnoid mater and runs between the free and the attached margins of the tentorium cerebelli before piercing the inner layer of the dura mater. It grooves the lateral side of the posterior clinoid process of the sphenoid bone, pierces the roof of the cavernous venous sinus and runs forwards in the upper part of its lateral wall: the trochlear nerve is here inferior to it. The oculomotor nerve divides into upper and lower divisions which enter the orbit through the superior orbital fissure (Fig 20). The superior division supplies the levator palpebrae superioris and superior rectus muscles: the inferior divison innervates the medial rectus, inferior rectus and inferior oblique muscles: the branch to the last muscle sends a twig to the ciliary ganglion.

DEEP CENTRAL CONNECTIONS See Chapter 6.

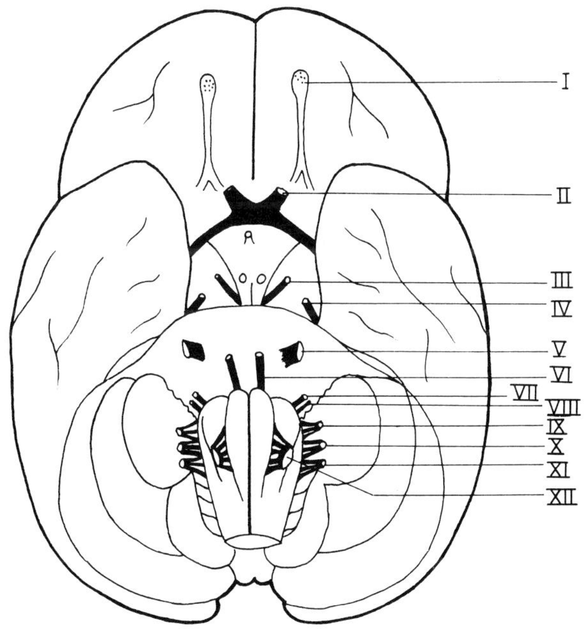

Fig 19 The origin of the cranial nerves.

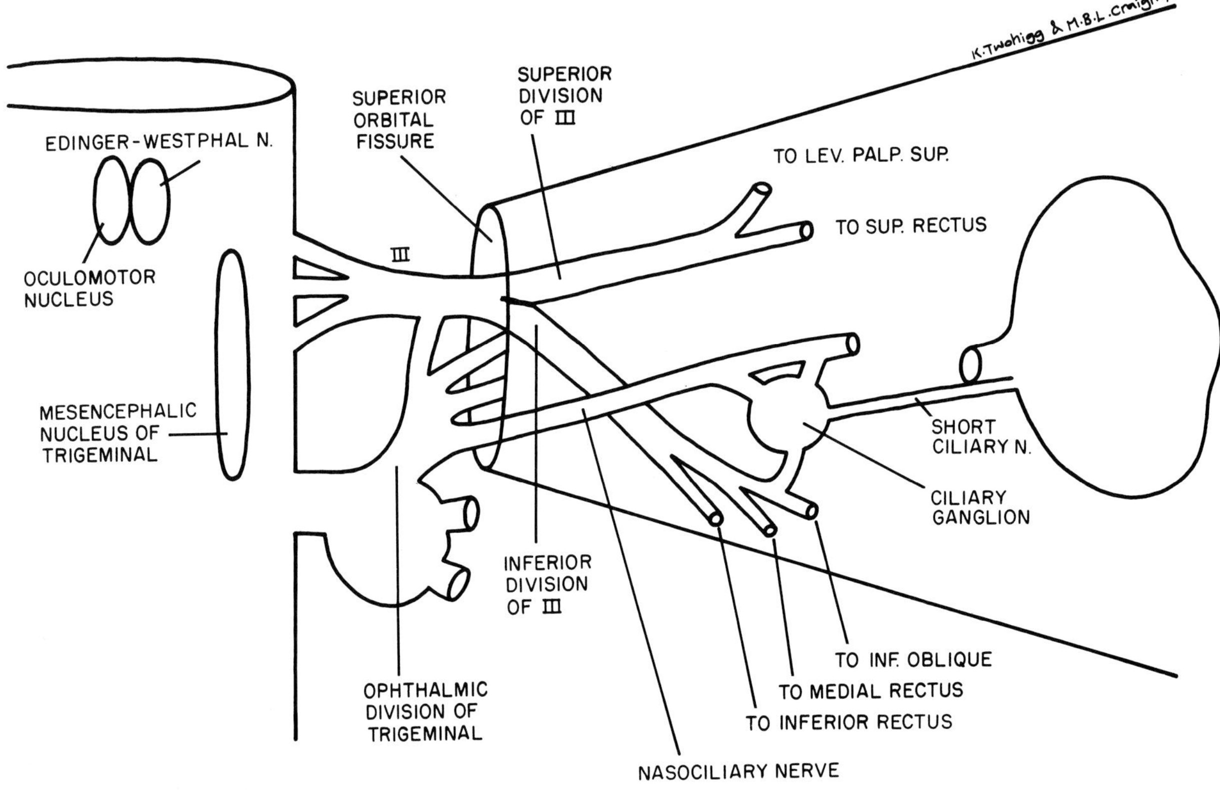

Fig 20   The distribution of the oculomotor nerve.

NUCLEAR CONNECTIONS

General somatic efferent component (Fig 21)

The oculomotor nucleus is the most cranial member of the general somatic efferent nuclei of the brain stem. The lower motor neurones in the nucleus supply:

(i)   levator palpebrae superioris
(ii) superior rectus
(iii) medial rectus   } extrinsic ocular muscles
(iv) inferior rectus
(v)   inferior oblique

General visceral efferent component (Fig 22)

The *Edinger-Westphal* nucleus is the isolated cranial end of the general visceral efferent column. The parasympathetic fibres from the nerve cells in the nucleus pass into the inferior division of the oculomotor nerve, then into its branch to the inferior oblique muscle and finally into the twig from this branch to the ciliary ganglion. The fibres synapse in the ganglion: post ganglionic fibres leave the ganglion in the short ciliary nerves, and so reach the back of the eyeball. The postganglionic parasympathetic fibres supply the smooth muscle of the ciliary body and of the sphincter pupillae.

General somatic afferent component (Fig 23)

The proprioceptive fibres from those extrinsic ocular muscles supplied by the oculomotor nerve (ie. all except

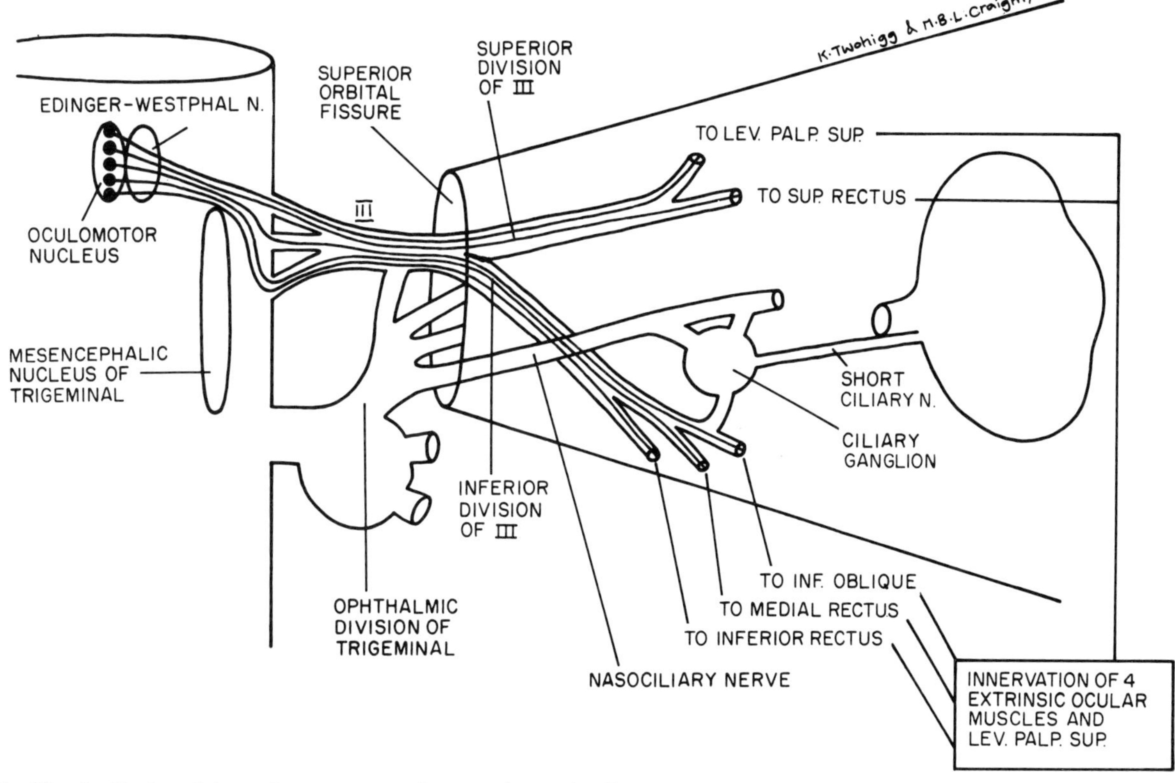

Fig 21 The distribution of the oculomotor nerve: the general somatic efferent component.

the lateral rectus and the superior oblique) are thought to be relayed in the *mesencephalic nucleus of the trigeminal nerve*. The afferents from the muscles pass in the oculomotor nerve as far as the cavernous sinus, where it is believed they join the ophthalmic division of the trigeminal nerve in a nerve of communication between them: they enter the brain stem in the sensory root of the trigeminal nerve. The axons of the cells in the mesencephalic nucleus of the trigeminal nerve relay in turn on the oculomotor nucleus (Fig 23).

The nuclear connections of the oculomotor nerve are summarised diagramatically in Figure 24.

DAMAGE TO THE OCULOMOTOR NERVE

The syndrome consequent upon division of the oculomotor nerve is as follows:

1 Paralysis of levator palpebrae superioris leads to *ptosis* (drooping of the upper eyelid).
2 Diplopia (double vision) when the lid is held up.
3 Paralysis of the superior, medial and inferior rectus muscles and the inferior oblique causes the eyeball to be deviated downwards and outwards and slight eyeball prominence (*proptosis*). The eyeball cannot be moved in any direction except laterally or downwards and outwards.
4 Paralysis of the smooth muscle of sphincter pupillae results in:
    (a) pupillary dilatation
    (b) loss of pupillary contraction on exposure to light.
5 Paralysis of the ciliary muscle leads to loss of power of accommodation.

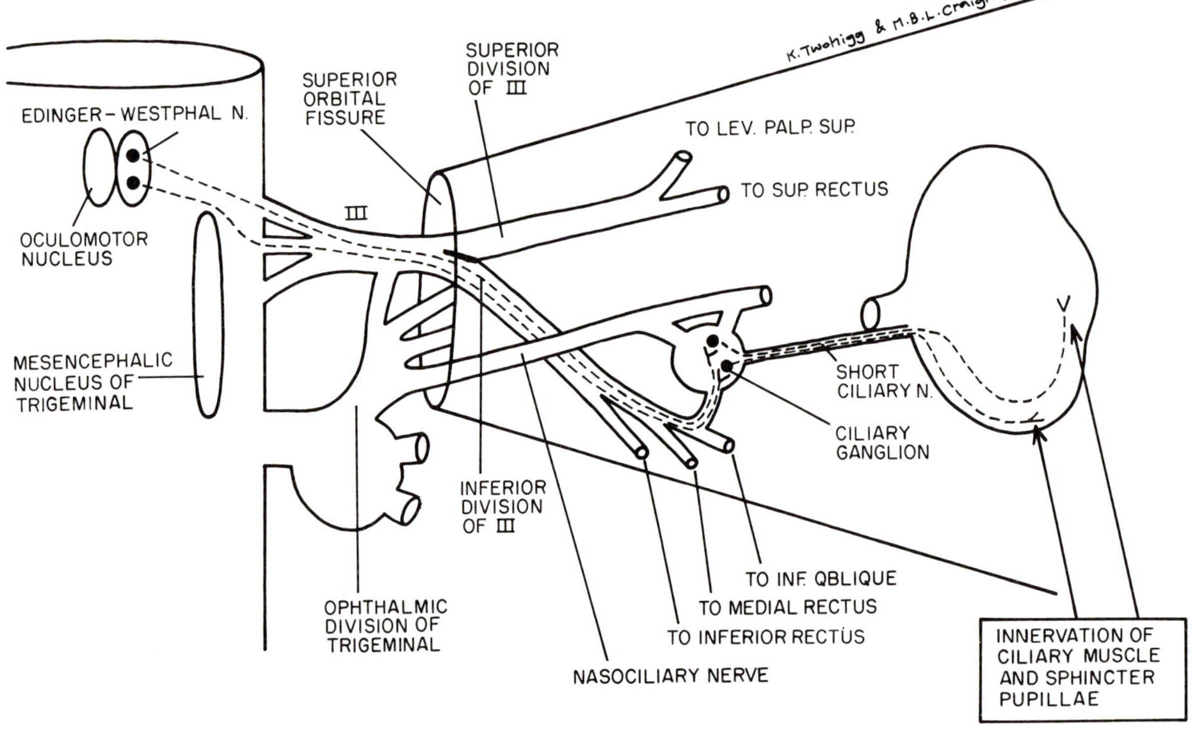

Fig 22   The distribution of the oculomotor nerve: the general visceral efferent component.

SITES OF LESION

1   *In the brain stem*

(a) Multiple sclerosis
(b) Poliomyelitis
(c) Gliomata of the brain stem
(d) Vascular lesions of the brain stem
(e) Wernick's encephalopathy

2   *In the basilar area*

(a) Aneurysm of the basilar artery
(b) Guillain-Barré syndrome
(c) Basal meningitis
(d) Neoplastic extensions from nasopharynx and paranasal air sinuses
(e) Sarcoid

(f) Herpes zoster
(g) Fractures

3   *In the area of the cavernous sinus*

(a) Cavernous sinus thrombosis
(b) Intrasellar tumours
(c) Aneurysm of the intracavernous part of the internal carotid artery
(d) Aneurysm of the posterior communicating artery
(e) Temporal lobe displacement causing stretching of the nerve over the edge of the tentorium cerebelli

4   *In the orbit*

(a) Tumours (meningiomata, haematomata or gliomata or carcinomata) behind the eyeball

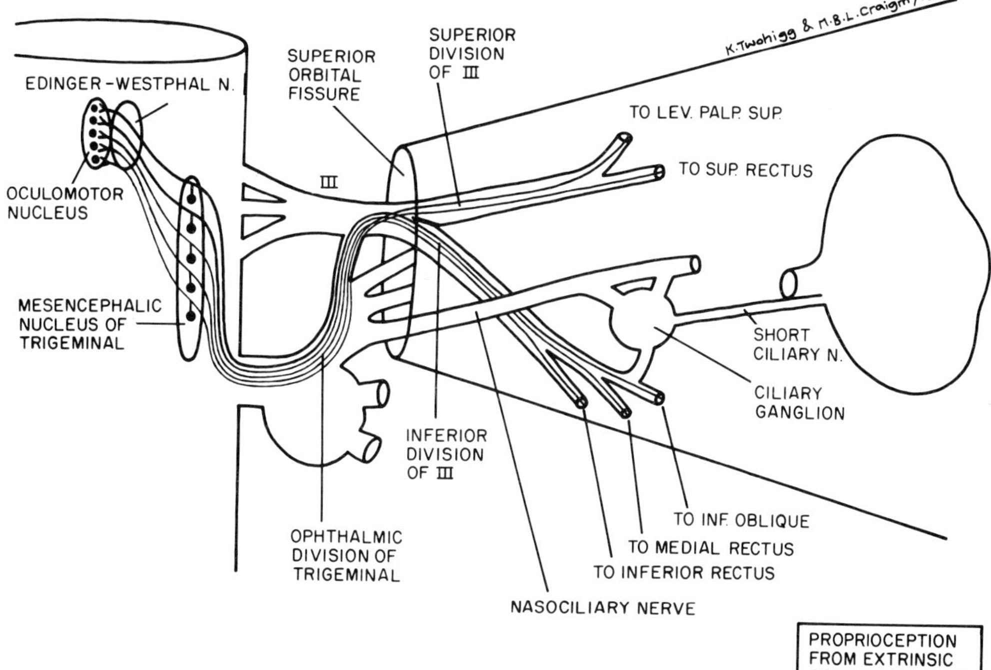

Fig 23 The distribution of the oculomotor nerve: the general somatic afferent component.

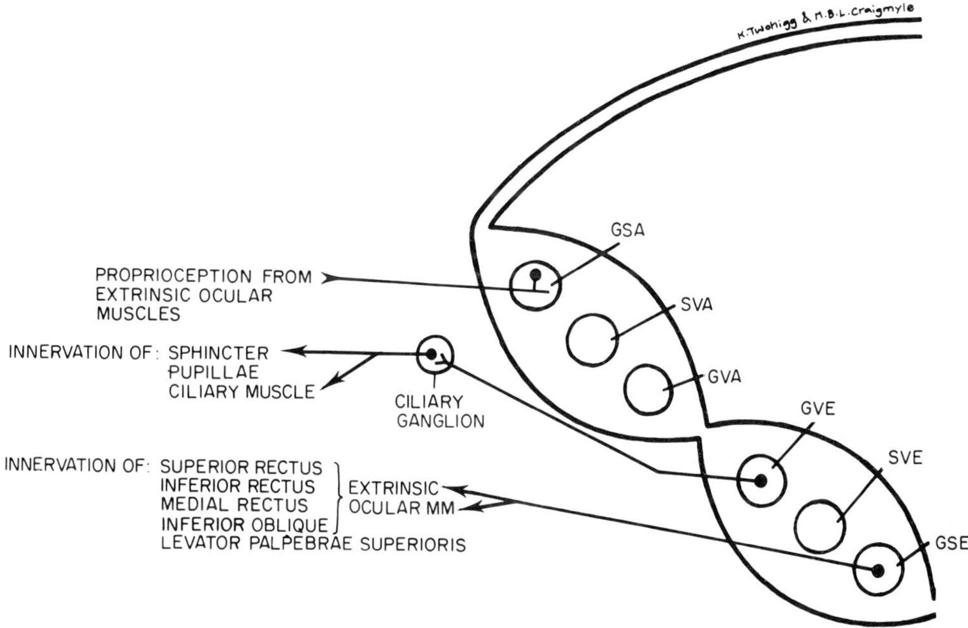

Fig 24 Summary of the nuclear connections of the oculomotor nerve.

8

THE TROCHLEAR NERVE

ORIGIN, COURSE AND DISTRIBUTION (Figs 19 and 25)

The trochlear nerve is unique in that it emerges from the dorsal aspect of the brain stem. The (GSE) fibres from opposite trochlear nuclei decussate in the superior medullary velum and, having crossed the midline, emerge from the velum just caudal to the inferior colliculus. The nerve turns round the basis pedunculi and passes between the posterior cerebral and superior cerebellar arteries. It pierces the dura mater at the free edge of the tentorum cerebelli and runs along the lateral wall of the cavernous sinus lying between the oculomotor nerve above and the ophthalmic division of the trigeminal nerve below. It crosses over the oculomotor nerve near the front of the cavernous sinus. It enters the orbit through the superior orbital fissure and passes above the common tendinous ring of origin of the rectus muscles. After crossing over levator palpebrae superioris, the nerve terminates by entering the superior oblique muscle from its orbital aspect.

DEEP CENTRAL CONNECTIONS These are summarised in Chapter 6

NUCLEAR CONNECTIONS OF THE TROCHLEAR NERVE

General somatic efferent component: *the trochlear nucleus* (Fig 26)

This nucleus lies in the floor of the central grey matter of the mid-brain at the level of the inferior colliculus. The fibres derived from this nucleus supply the superior oblique muscle.

General somatic afferent component: *the mesencephalic nucleus of the trigeminal nerve* (Fig 27)

The proprioceptive fibres from the superior oblique muscle are distal processes of the pseudo-unipolar nerve cells in the mesencephalic nucleus and whose central processes end in the trochlear nucleus. The route by which the fibres reach the brain stem is either via the trochlear nerve throughout or, more likely, via the trochlear nerve as far as the cavernous sinus and thereafter via the ophthalmic division of the trigeminal nerve, with which the trochlear nerve here com-

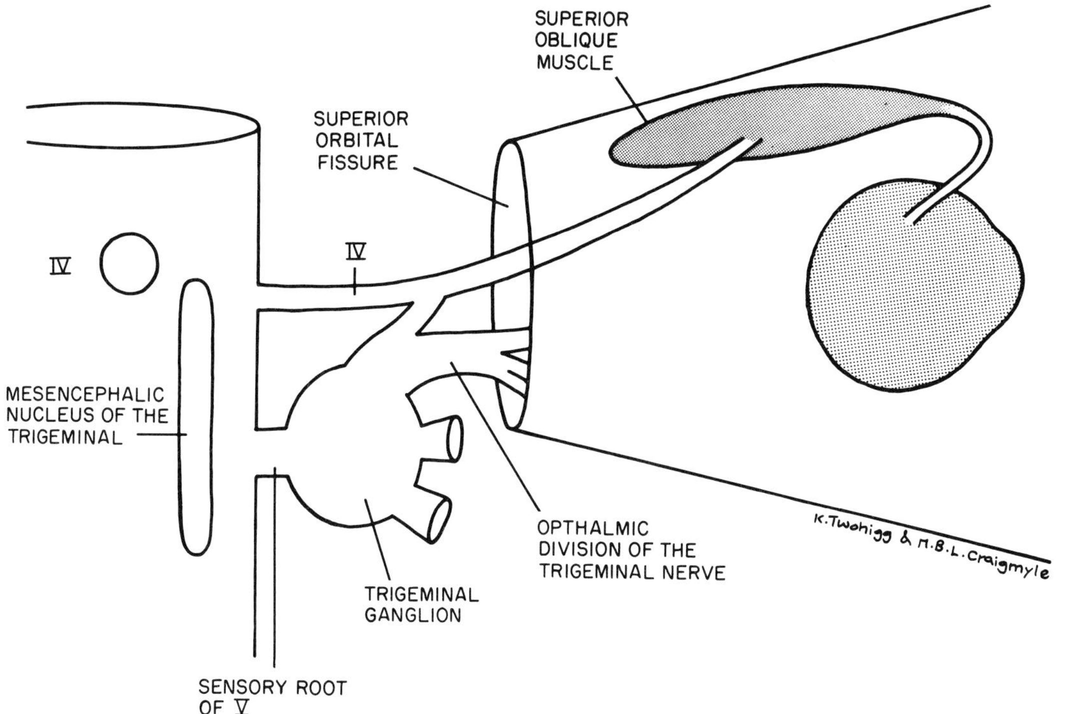

Fig 25 The distribution of the trochlear nerve.

municates, and the sensory root of the trigeminal nerve.

The nuclear connections of the trochlear nerve are summarised in Figure 28.

LESIONS OF THE TROCHLEAR NERVE

Paralysis of the superior oblique muscle leads to diplopia (double vision) on looking down and strabismus (squint). The squint is not obvious and the condition is a difficult one to detect. The patient may carry his head with a tilt to the affected side: in children this may be mistaken for torticollis. The only disability is an inability to depress the adducted eye on the affected side.

SITES OF LESION

1 *In the brain stem*

(a) Mutliple sclerosis

(b) Poliomyelitis

(c) Glioma

(d) Vascular lesions

(e) Wernick's encephalopathy

2 *In the basilar area*

(a) Aneurysm of the basilar artery

(b) Guillain-Barré syndrome

(c) Basal meningitis

(d) Neoplasia of nasopharynx or paranasal air sinuses

(e) Sarcoid

(f) Herpes zoster

(g) Fractures

3 *In the area of the cavernous sinus*

(a) Cavernous sinus thrombosis

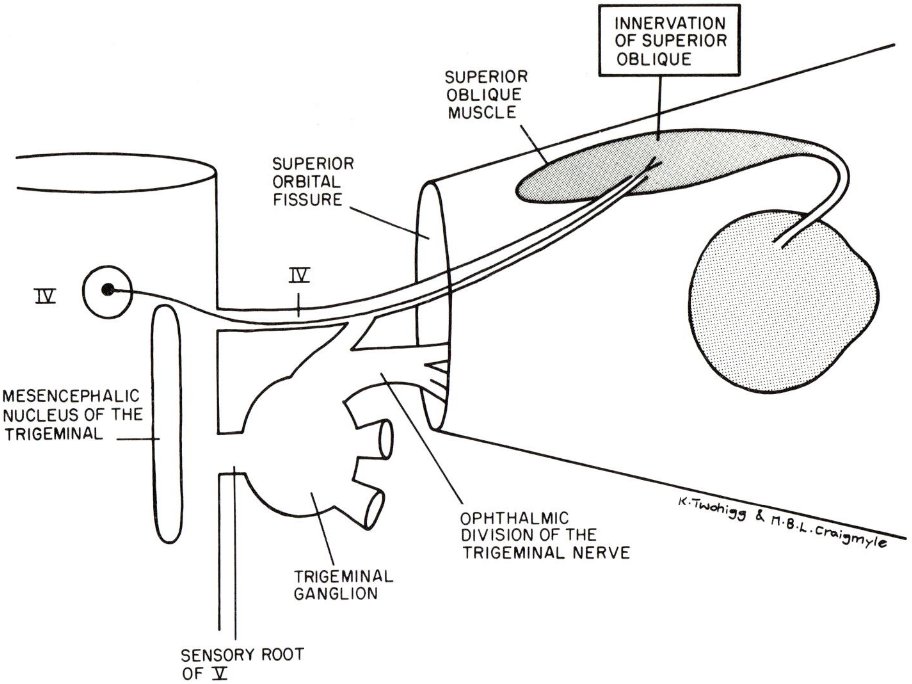

Fig 26   The distribution of the trochlear nerve: the general somatic efferent component.

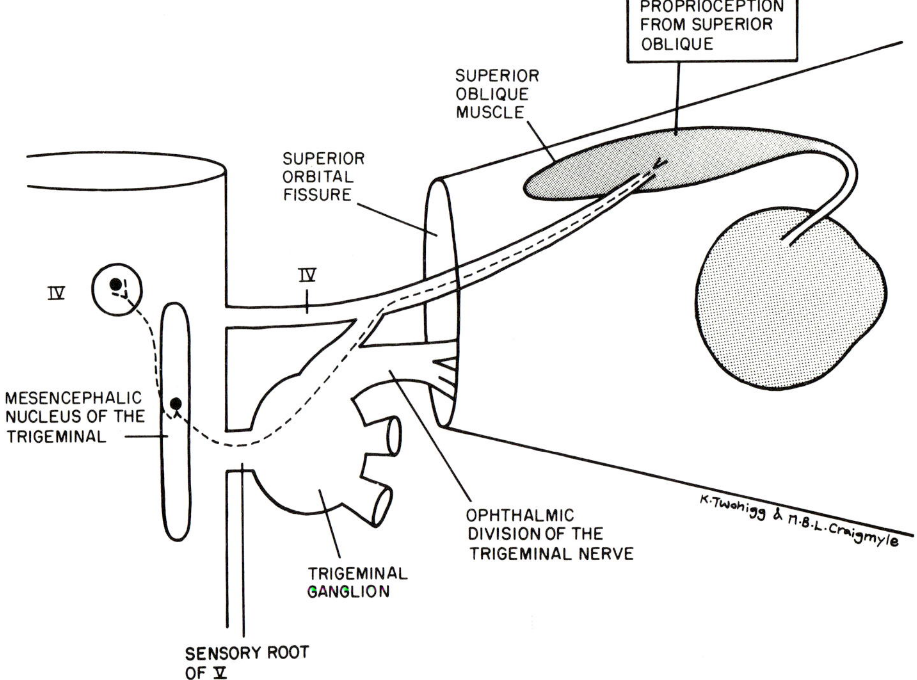

Fig 27   The distribution of the trochlear nerve: the general somatic afferent component.

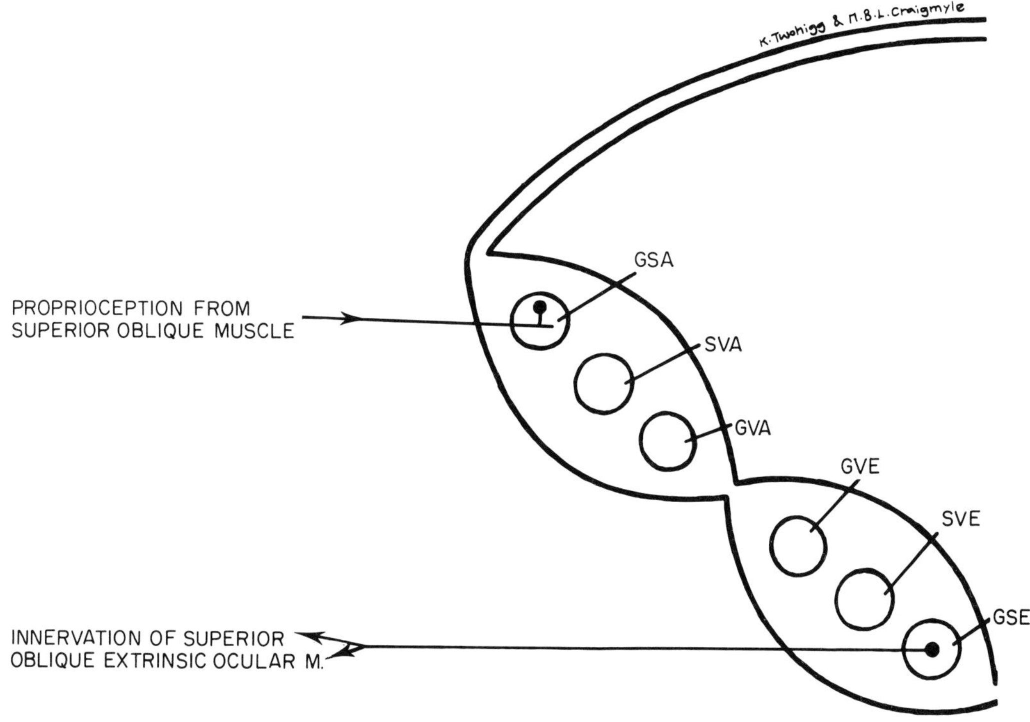

Fig 28 Summary of the nuclear connections of the trochlear nerve.

(b) Intrasellar tumours

(c) Aneurysm of the intracavernous part of the internal carotid artery

(d) Aneurysm of the posterior communicating artery

(e) Temporal lobe enlargement or displacement causing the nerve to be stretched over the edge of the tentorium cerebelli

4 In the orbit

(a) Simple tumours behind the eyeball such as meningiomata, gliomata or haemangiomata

(b) Retro-orbital carcinoma

9

THE TRIGEMINAL NERVE AND THE CRANIAL PARASYMPATHETIC GANGLIA

ORIGIN, COURSE AND DISTRIBUTION OF THE TRIGEMINAL NERVE

This is the largest of the cranial nerves and takes origin from the middle of the pons by two roots, a large sensory and a small motor root (Fig 19). The sensory (GSA) root is composed of the centrally-directed processes of the pseudo-unipolar nerve cells in the trigeminal ganglion. The motor (SVE) root arises from the pons postero-superior to the sensory root. The distally-running processes of the pseudo-unipolar nerve cells in the ganglion form the ophthalmic and maxillary divisions of the trigeminal nerve and also the sensory component of the mandibular division: the motor root passes under the ganglion, and leaves the skull via the foramen ovale, in company with the sensory component. The two unite immediately below the skull in the infratemporal fossa to form the mandibular division proper (Fig 29).

The trigeminal ganglion is large, flattened and semilunar in shape: it occupies a shallow bony concavity on the dorsum of the apex of the petrous portion of the temporal bone. It lies in the cavum trigeminale, a pouch-like extension of the dura mater of the posterial cranial fossa into the middle cranial fossa.

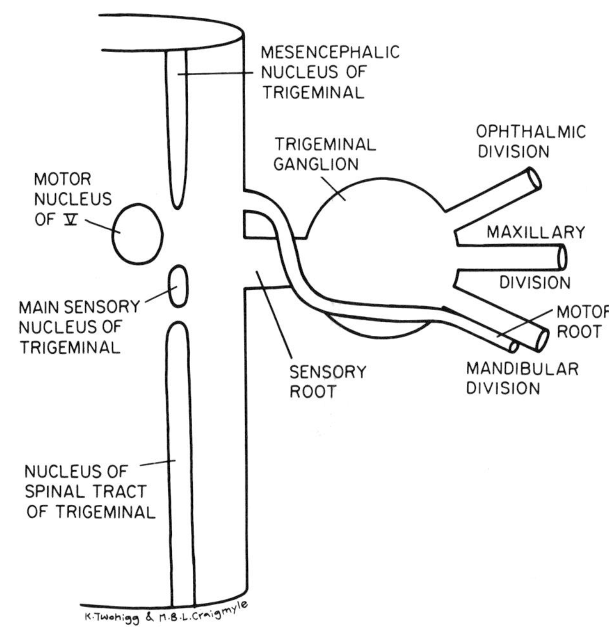

Fig 29 The distribution of the trigeminal nerve.

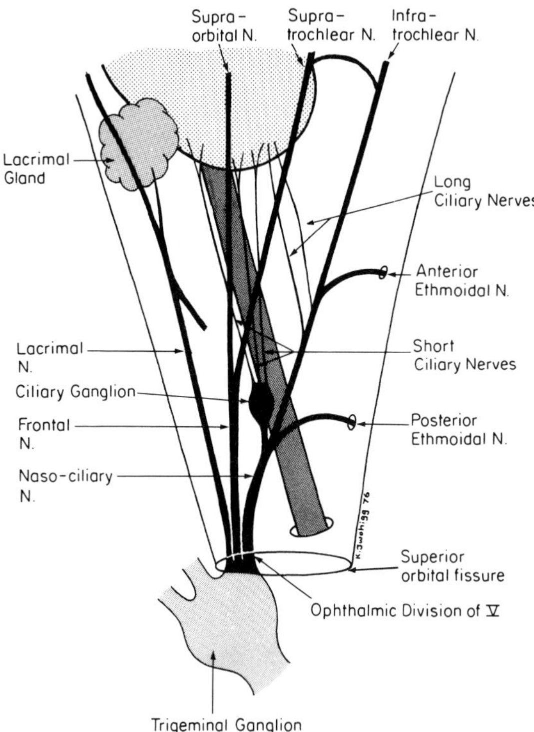

Fig 30   The ophthalmic division of the trigeminal nerve.

THE OPHTHALMIC DIVISION OF THE TRIGEMINAL NERVE (Fig 30)

This, the smallest of the three divisions, runs forwards from the trigeminal ganglion in the lateral wall of the cavernous sinus accompanied by the oculomotor and trochlear nerves above and the abducent and maxillary nerves below. It here communicates with the first three of these nerves. The ophthalmic nerve divides, just behind the superior orbital fissure, into three terminal branches: the lacrimal, frontal and nasociliary nerves.

The lacrimal nerve

This nerve passes through the most lateral part of the superior orbital fissure to enter the cavity of the orbit. It runs along the lateral wall of the orbit above the lateral rectus muscle, and enters the lacrimal gland, to which it gives branches. After emerging from the gland it enters the upper eyelid from its lateral aspect. It is distributed to the gland, to the conjunctiva and to the skin of the upper eyelid. In its passage through the orbit it is joined by a twig from the zygomatic branch of the maxillary nerve: this conveys (GVE) parasympathetic postganglionic secretomotor fibres from the pterygopalatine ganglion to the lacrimal gland myoepithelium (Fig 33).

The frontal nerve

This nerve passes through the superior orbital fissure to reach the orbit: it runs along the orbital roof, and crosses over the levator palpebrae superioris muscle from lateral to medial. About mid-orbit it divides into a small medial supratrochlear branch and a large lateral supraorbital branch. The *supratrochlear nerve* runs to the medial angle of the eye where it communicates with the infra-trochlear branch of the nasociliary nerve. After passing over the pulley of the superior oblique muscle it reaches and supplies the skin of the medial part of the forehead, of the root of the nose, and of the medial part of the upper eyelid and the associated conjunctiva. The *supra-orbital nerve* runs forwards to the supra-orbital notch (of the frontal bone) on the upper rim of the orbital margin. It divides into branches which supply the mucosa of the frontal air sinus and the skin of the upper eyelid. The largest branch ascends over the forehead deep to the frontal belly of the occipitofrontalis muscle to become cutaneous to that part of the scalp anterior to the lambdoid suture.

The nasociliary nerve

This passes through the superior orbital fissure to enter the cavity of the orbit. It lies at first between the upper and lower divisions of the oculomotor nerve. It runs anteromedially, and crosses the optic nerve. It gives off a small twig (sensory root) to the ciliary ganglion and a *posterior ethmoidal* branch. The latter enters the posterior ethmoidal canal on the medial wall of the orbit to reach and supply the mucosa of the sphenoidal and posterior ethmoidal air sinuses. The nasociliary nerve then gives off two *long ciliary nerves* which pass to the eyeball to be sensory to the cornea, iris and ciliary body before dividing into its terminal branches, the anterior ethmoidal and infratrochlear nerves. The *anterior*

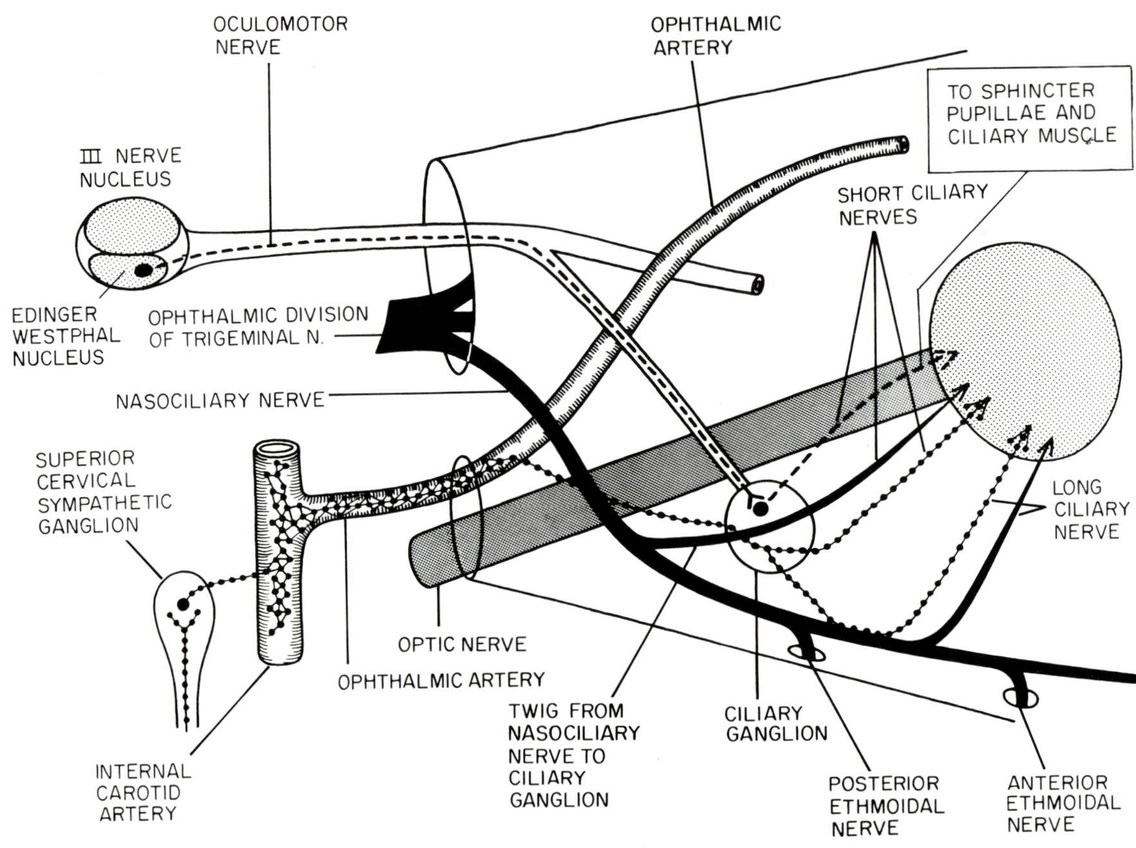

Fig 31   The ciliary ganglion and its connections.

ethmoidal nerve enters the anterior ethmoidal canal on the medial wall of the orbit, and so reaches the anterior cranial fossa at the lateral edge of the cribriform plate of the ethmoid bone. It runs medially across the plate to reach the crista galli before descending through the plate to reach the roof of the nasal cavity. It here divides into a small medial internal nasal branch distributed to the mucosa of the anterosuperior part of the nasal septum, and a larger lateral internal nasal branch. The latter supplies the mucosa of the anterosuperior part of the nasal septum before passing between the nasal bone and the upper lateral nasal cartilage to reach and supply the skin of the ala, the vestibule, and the tip of the nose. The *infratrochlear branch* runs forward on the medial orbital wall above the medial rectus muscle. Near the pulley of

the superior oblique muscle it communicates with the supratrochlear nerve. It is distributed to the conjunctiva, to the mucosa of the lacrimal sac and issues from the medial margin of the orbit to reach the skin of both eyelids and of the side of the nose.

THE CILIARY GANGLION AND ITS CONNECTIONS (Figs 30 and 31)

The ciliary ganglion is small, flattened, and of pin-head size. It lies near the apex of the orbit between the optic nerve and the lateral rectus muscle. It receives three *roots* (motor, sensory and sympathetic) which enter it from behind and gives rise to between six and ten branches, the *short ciliary nerves*, which pass from the front

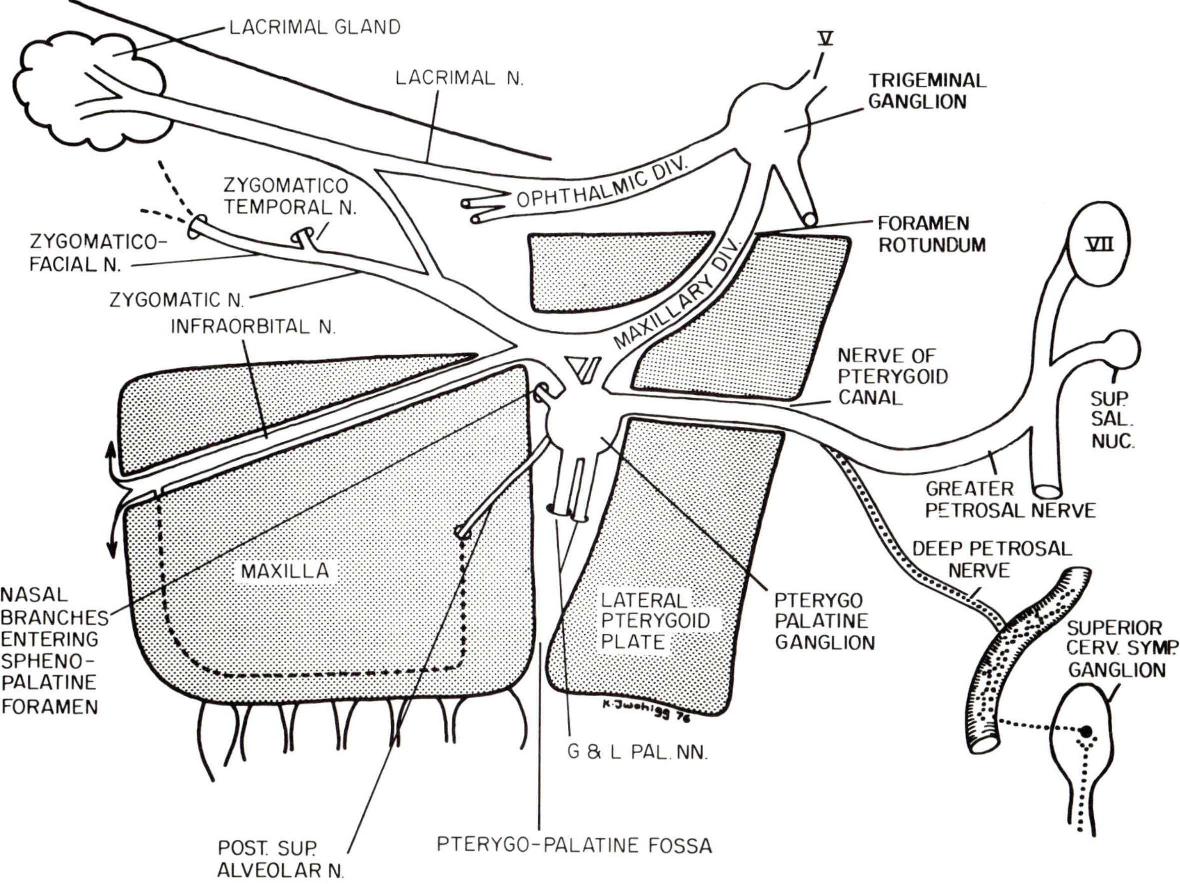

Fig 32   The distribution of the maxillary division of the trigeminal nerve.

of the ganglion to the back of the eyeball in two sets, one above and one below the optic nerve. They pierce the sclera around the exit of the optic nerve, and pass to the front of the eyeball deep to the sclera.

The *motor root* (dashes in Fig 31) alone relays within the ganglion. It arises from the branch of the oculomotor nerve to the inferior oblique muscle. It conveys preganglionic parasympathetic (GVE) fibres from the Edinger-Westphal nucleus. After a relay in the ganglion, postganglionic fibres pass in the short ciliary nerves to the smooth muscle of the ciliary body and sphincter pupillae.

The *sensory root* (black line in Fig 31) is a ramus communicans from the nasociliary nerve to the ganglion: its contained fibres (GSA) pass through the ganglion without interruption and enter the short ciliary nerves. They are sensory to the cornea, iris and ciliary body.

The *sympathetic root* (dotted line in Fig 31) is combined not infrequently with the sensory root. It consists of a ramus communicans from the plexus on the ophthalmic artery to the ganglion. It contains postganglionic sympathetic (GVE) fibres from the superior cervical sympathetic ganglion via the plexus on the internal carotid artery. The fibres pass through the ganglion without interruption, enter the short ciliary nerves and are vasomotor to the blood vessels of the choroid.

THE MAXILLARY DIVISION (Fig 32)

This division runs forwards from the trigeminal ganglion in the lower part of the lateral wall of the cavernous sinus beow the abducent nerve. It leaves the middle cranial fossa via the foramen rotundum which leads it into the superior part of the pterygopalatine fossa. After rounding the lateral side of the orbital process of the palatine bone, it enters the orbit through the inferior orbital fissure. It runs forward in the infra-orbital groove on the orbital floor, and is now known as the *infra-orbital nerve*. It passes from the infra-orbital groove into the infra-orbital canal and emerges on the cheek through the infra-orbital foramen of the maxilla. It is distributed to the skin of the lower eyelid, of the side of the nose, of the cheek and upper lip and to the mucosa of the upper lip and cheek.

Branches of the maxillary nerve

1   *In the middle cranial fossa: a meningeal branch (not shown in Fig 32)*

2   *In the pterygopalatine fossa:*

    (i)   direct branches
        (a)   the ganglionic branches to the pterygo-palatine ganglion
        (b)   the zygomatic nerve
        (c)   the posterior superior alveolar nerve
    (ii) indirect branches via the pterygopalatine ganglion
        (a)   nasal branches
        (b)   palatine branches
        (c)   pharyngeal branch (not shown in Fig 32)

3   *In the infra-orbital canal*

        (a)   the middle superior alveolar nerve (not shown)
        (b)   the anterior superior alveolar nerve

4   *On the face*

        (a)   palpebral branches
        (b)   nasal branches
        (c)   labial branches

The *meningeal branch* is given off in the middle cranial fossa: it supplies the dura mater of the middle and anterior cranial fossae (it is not shown in Fig 32).

The *ganglionic branches* consist (usually) of two branches to the pterygopalatine ganglion, which constitute its sensory root.

The *zygomatic nerve* arises in the pterygopalatine fossa, enters the orbit through the inferior orbital fissure, and runs along the lateral orbital wall. It gives off a communicating branch to the lacrimal nerve before terminating in *zygomaticotemporal* and *zygomatico-facial branches*: these pass through canals in the zygomatic bone to emerge from the zygomaticotemporal and zygomaticofacial foramina of the same bone. The first nerve is distributed to the skin of the temple and the second to the skin of the malar eminence. (The communicating branch of the zygomatic nerve to the lacrimal nerve conveys (GVE) postganglionic parasympathetic secretomotor fibres from the pterygo-palatine ganglion to the lacrimal gland myoepithelium.)

The *posterior superior alveolar nerve* arises from the maxillary nerve in the pterygopalatine fossa, and passes laterally through the pterygomaxillary fissure to reach the infratemporal fossa. It then enters the posterior dental canal on the posterolateral aspect of the maxilla by which means it reaches and supplies the upper molar and premolar teeth and adjacent gums, and the mucosa of the maxillary sinus. It continues forward to join the anterior superior dental nerve and so complete the superior alveolar nervous loop.

The *middle superior alveolar nerve*, rarely present, arises from the maxillary nerve or its infra-orbital continuation. It descends in the mucosa of the lateral wall of the maxillary sinus to supply the upper premolar teeth. It communicates with both the anterior superior and posterior superior alveolar nerves (it is not shown in Fig 32).

The *anterior superior alveolar nerve* takes origin from the infra-orbital nerve while it is running in the infra-orbital canal. The nerve descends in a bony canal anterior to the maxillary antrum to reach and supply the upper incisor and canine teeth and adjacent gums. It communicates with the middle superior alveolar nerve when present, and when this nerve is absent, with the posterior superior alveolar nerve. It gives off a small *nasal* branch which passes through a bony canal to reach the mucosa of the floor and of the anterior part of the lateral wall of the nasal cavity (this branch is not shown in Fig 32).

The *greater palatine nerve* arises indirectly from the maxillary nerve via the pterygopalatine ganglion. It descends in the greater palatine canal between the maxilla and the perpendicular plate of the palatine bone and emerges on the bony palate through the greater palatine foramen. It runs forward on the underside of the hard palate in a bony groove and is distributed to the mucosa (with its contained glands) of the hard palate. It subserves ordinary sensation and taste. Within the greater palatine canal it gives off nasal branches which pass through the perpendicular plate of the palatine bone to supply the mucous membrane of the lateral nasal wall over the middle meatus, the inferior concha and the inferior meatus (these are not shown in Fig 32).

The *lesser palatine nerves*, usually two in number, also arise from the maxillary nerve only indirectly via the pterygopalatine ganglion. They descend in the greater palatine canal but issue on the hard palate through the lesser palatine foramina. They are distributed to the mucosa of the soft palate (including the uvula) and the tonsil. Like the greater palatine nerve, they subserve ordinary sensation and taste. (The SVA fibres conveying taste sensation from the palate pass in the greater and lesser palatine nerves to the pterygopalatine ganglion, through which they pass without interruption, to run in the nerve of the pterygoid canal and the greater petrosal branch of the facial nerve: the fibres are the dendrites of the pseudo-unipolar neurones of the facial ganglion (Fig 16). The axons of the same cells pass into the brain stem in the sensory root of the facial nerve and terminate in the upper part of the nucleus of the tractus solitarius.)

The *nasal branches* of the maxillary nerve also originate from the pterygopalatine ganglion. They enter the spheno-ethmoidal recess of the nasal cavity by passing through the sphenopalatine foramen, and divide into two sets. One set, the lateral posterior superior, supplies the mucosa of the lateral nasal wall over the superior and middle conchae and also the mucosa of the posterior ethmoidal air sinuses. The second group, the medial posterior superior, runs across the roof of the nasal cavity, supplying it, to reach the nasal septum, which is also supplied by this group: one member, the nasopalatine nerve, runs obliquely downwards and forwards on the septum, passes through the incisive foramen and supplies the mucosa of the front of the hard palate.

The *pharyngeal branch* of the maxillary nerve arises from the back of the pterygopalatine ganglion and passes backwards through the palatinovaginal canal to reach and be distributed to the mucosa of the nasopharynx behind the orifice of the pharyngotympanic tube. It is not shown in Figure 32.

THE PTERYGOPALATINE GANGLION AND ITS CONNECTIONS (Figs 16, 33 and 48)

The ganglion receives motor, sensory and sympathetic roots. The sensory roots are usually two in number and their origin from the maxillary nerve has been described earlier in the chapter. The motor and sympathetic roots arrive, in combination, as the nerve of the pterygoid canal, which joins the posterior aspect of the ganglion (Fig 33).

The *motor root* (interrupted dashes, Fig 33) is composed of preganglionic parasympathetic fibres from the superior salivary (GVE) nucleus. These pass into the facial nerve via its motor root and leave the nerve in its greater petrosal branch: this joins the deep petrosal nerve to form the nerve of the pterygoid canal. The fibres synapse in the ganglion. The postganglionic parasympathetic fibres are secreto-motor in function, and pass in the branches of the ganglion to supply the myoepithelium of:

1 the salivary glands of the palate in the greater and lesser palatine nerves;
2 the salivary glands of the nasal cavity in the nasal branches of the ganglion; and
3 the lacrimal (salivary) gland in a branch of the ganglion to the zygomatic nerve and thence, through a communicating branch, the lacrimal nerve.

The *sympathetic root* (dotted line, Fig 33) is composed of post-ganglionic sympathetic fibres from the superior

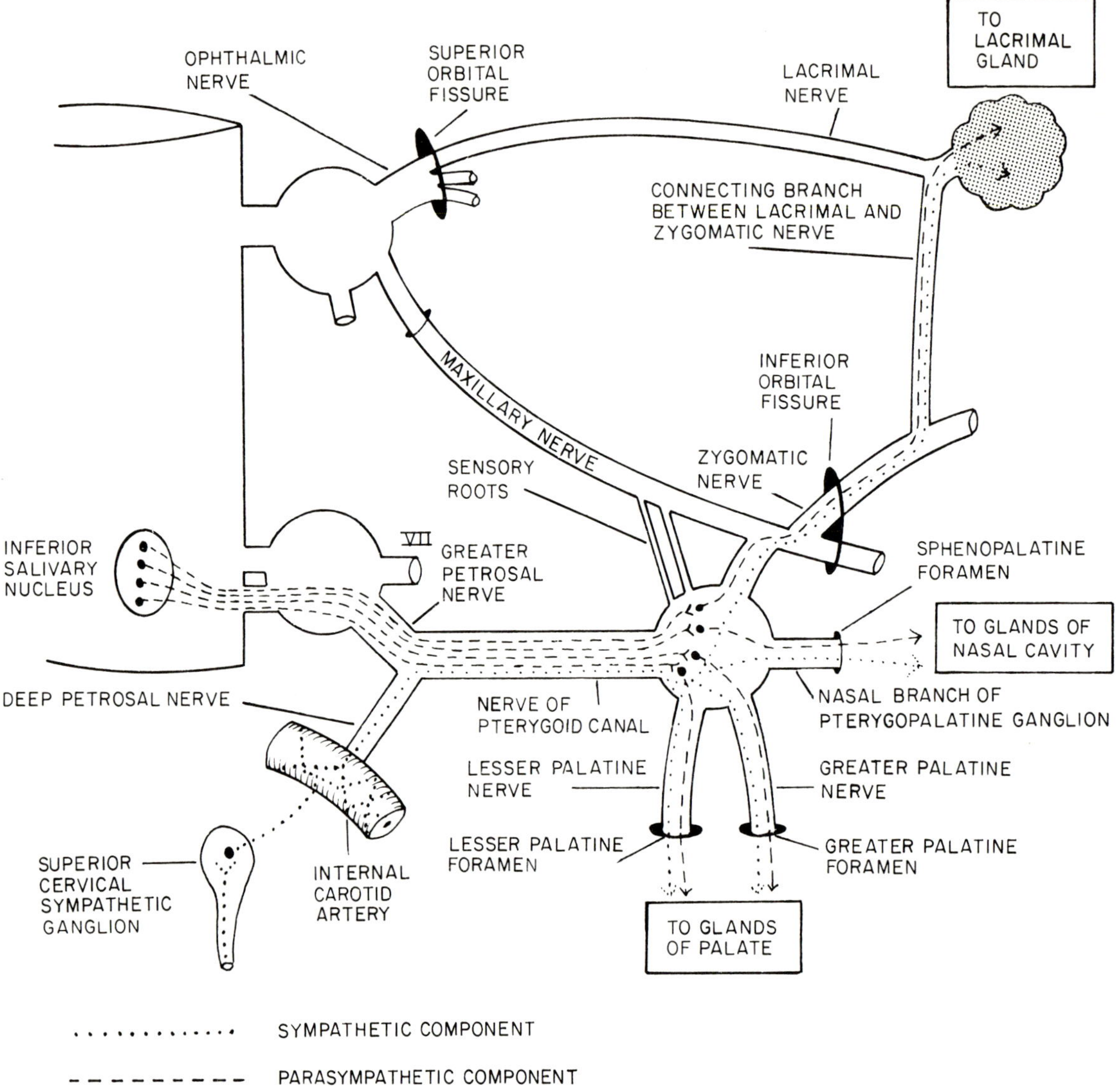

Fig 33 The connections of the pterygopalatine ganglion.

cervical sympathetic ganglion. These form a plexus on the internal carotid artery from which a twig, the deep petrosal nerve, passes into the pterygoid canal to join the greater petrosal nerve to form the nerve of the pterygoid canal. The sympathetic fibres pass through the ganglion without interruption and are distributed to (and are vasomotor to) the blood vessels of the nasal cavity, the palate, the pharynx and the lacrimal gland in the branches of the ganglion.

The *sensory root* is composed of branches (usually two) from the maxillary nerve to the ganglion: they contain GSA fibres which pass through the ganglion

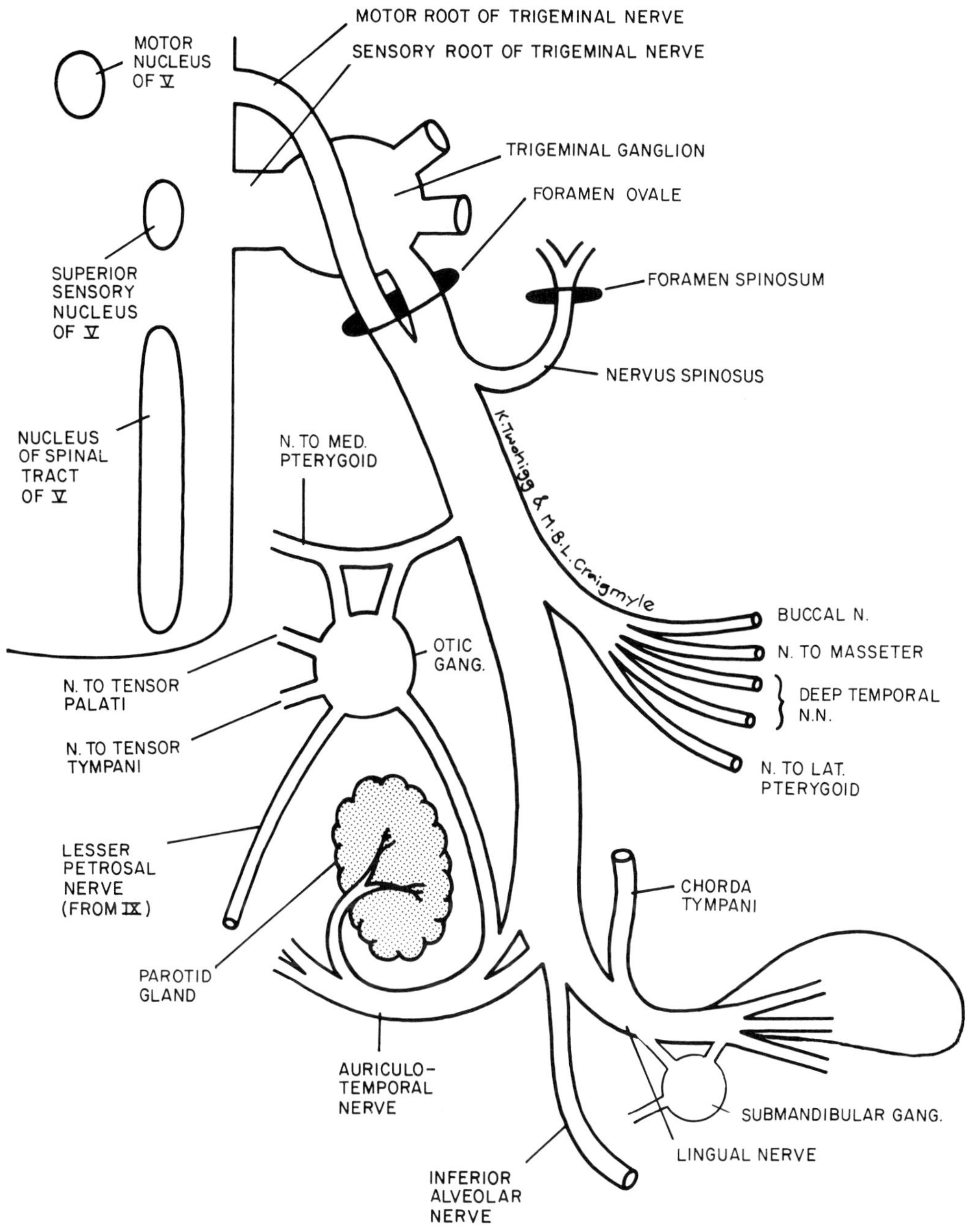

Fig 34 The distribution of the mandibular division of the trigeminal nerve.

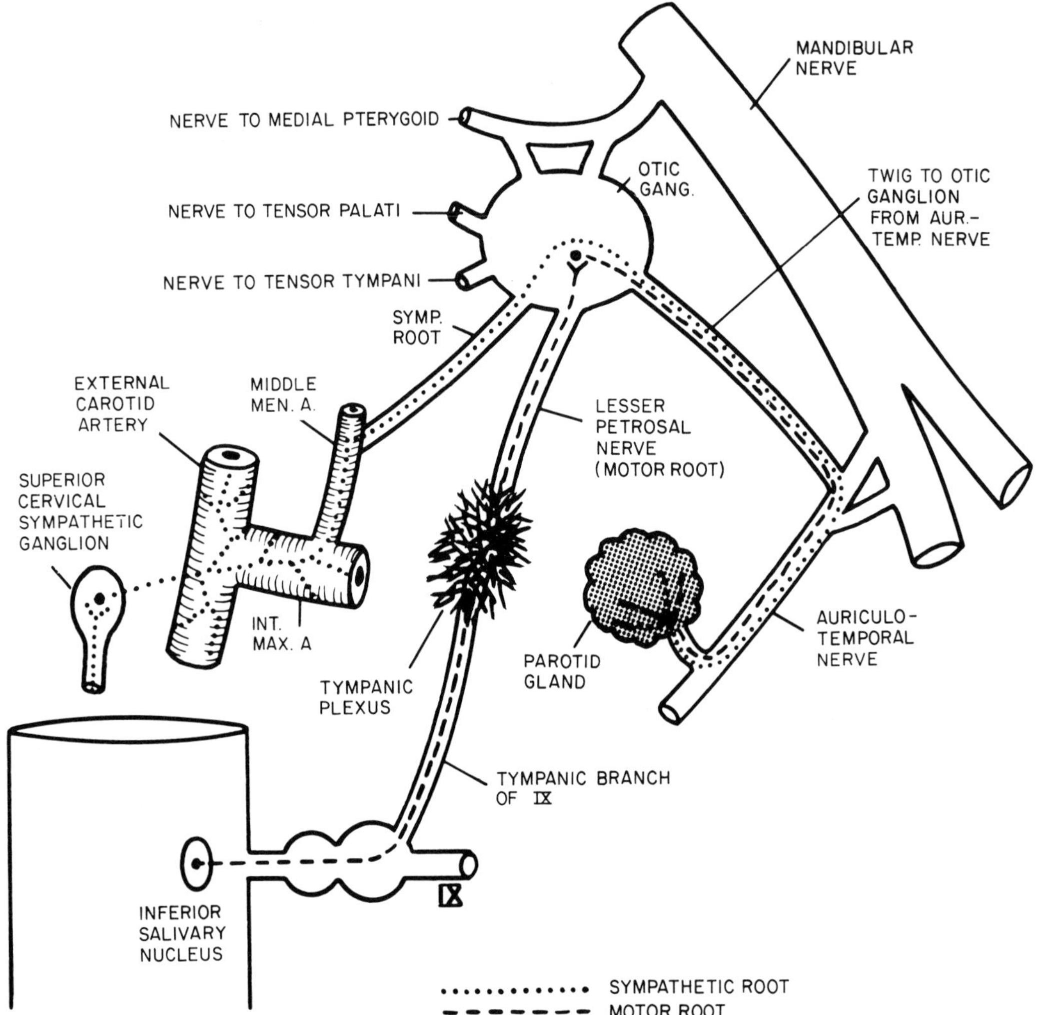

Fig 35   The connections of the otic ganglion.

without synapse and are sensory to the mucoperiosteum of the nasal cavity, pharynx and palate which they reach in the *branches of the ganglion*. These, the nasal, palatine and pharyngeal nerves, have been described earlier in the chapter.

THE MANDIBULAR DIVISION (Fig 34)

The *mandibular division* is the largest of the three divisions of the trigeminal nerve. It is formed in the infratemporal fossa just below the foramen ovale by the union of the motor root of the trigeminal nerve with the mandibular branch of the trigeminal ganglion, both of which pass through the foramen ovale. The nerve gives off, almost at once, two small branches, the meningeal branch (nervus spinosus) and the *nerve to the medial pterygoid muscle* before dividing into anterior and posterior divisions. From the posterior division arise the *lingual, inferior alveolar* and *auriculotemporal nerves*. From the anterior division arise the *buccal nerve* and the *nerve to the masseter* muscle, the *nerve to the lateral pterygoid* muscle and the two *deep temporal nerves* which supply the temporalis muscle.

The *nervous spinosus* passes through the foramen spinosum in the greater wing of the sphenoid bone to reach the floor of the middle cranial fossa: it is distributed to the dura mater of the middle and anterior cranial fossae and to the mucous membrane of the mastoid air cells.

The *nerve to the medial pterygoid* muscle is slender, and enters the muscle from its deep aspect. It is connected to the otic ganglion by one or two filaments.

THE OTIC GANGLION AND ITS CONNECTIONS
(Figs 35 and 53)

The otic ganglion is minute: it lies in the infratemporal fossa just below the foramen ovale. It is situated medial to the mandibular nerve and just behind the posterior edge of the medial pterygoid muscle. In common with all the cranial parasympathetic ganglia it has three roots (sensory, motor and sympathetic) and it possesses five branches, which are:

1 the nerve to the tensor palati muscle,
2 the nerve to the tensor tympani muscle,
3 a communicating branch to the auriculotemporal nerve,
4 a communicating branch to the chorda tympani nerve (not shown in Fig 35), and
5 a communicating branch to the nerve of the pterygoid canal (not shown in Fig 35).

The *motor root* (interrupted dashes, Fig 35) is the lesser petrosal nerve. It conveys preganglionic parasympathetic secretomotor fibres which arise in the inferior salivary (GVE) nucleus. The fibres pass into the glossopharyngeal nerve and leave it in its tympanic branch, which runs to the tympanic plexus on the promontory of the tympanum. The fibres leave the plexus in the lesser petrosal nerve, which after passing through a canal in the temporal bone, reaches the middle cranial fossa, passes through the foramen ovale and joins the otic ganglion. There the fibres relay before passing into the communicating branch of the ganglion with the auriculotemporal nerve. This nerve carries them to the parotid gland, to the myoepithelium of which they are distributed.

The *sympathetic root* is formed of postganglionic sympathetic fibres from the superior cervical sympathetic ganglion (dotted line in Fig 35). These pass to the plexus in the tunica adventitia of the external carotid artery and in turn its internal maxillary and middle meningeal branches. A twig from the last vessel to the ganglion is the sympathetic root: the contained fibres pass through the ganglion without interruption to reach the parotid gland via the twig from the ganglion to the auriculotemporal nerve. They are vasomotor in function.

The *sensory root* consists of fibres from the mandibular nerve via its branch to the medial pterygoid muscle. In the case of this ganglion, the term sensory is probably a misnomer since the trigeminal nerve fibres in this case are mostly motor (SVE) fibres from the motor nucleus of the nerve which pass through the ganglion without interruption to reach the tensor palati and tensor tympani muscles in the twigs from the ganglion to the muscle in question.

The *buccal nerve* arises from the anterior division of the mandibular nerve (Fig 34). It passes between the heads of the lateral pterygoid muscle and through or beneath the temporalis muscle and then issues from in front of the ramus of the mandible to reach and supply the mucosa and skin of the cheek.

The *auriculotemporal nerve* arises by two roots from the posterior division of the mandibular nerve (Fig 34). The middle meningeal artery passes between the two roots. The nerve passes between the neck of the mandible and the sphenomandibular ligament and behind the temporomandibular joint, to which it gives a twig. The nerve is here deep to the parotid gland, to which it gives several branches: it then ascends over the zygomatic arch to terminate in cutaneous branches to the temple. It also supplies the skin of the external acoustic meatus and tympanic membrane and the skin of the upper half of the pinna on its lateral aspect.

The *inferior alveolar nerve* is also a branch of the posterior division of the mandibular nerve (Fig 34). It descends under cover of the lateral pterygoid muscle to reach the interval between the ramus of the mandible and the medial pterygoid muscle. It gives off the *nerve to mylohyoid* which pierces the sphenomandibular ligament and runs in a groove on the medial surface of the ramus of the mandible to reach and supply the mylohyoid muscle and the anterior belly of the digastric muscle. The inferior alveolar nerve enters the mandibular foramen to run in the mandibular canal below the molar and premolar teeth, supplying them and the gum on either side. The nerve then divides into an incisive and a mental branch. The *incisive branch continues on in the mandibular canal, supplying the* ipsilateral canine tooth and the incisive teeth on both sides of the midline. The *mental branch* emerges through the mental foramen in the body of the mandible to reach the skin of the chin and the mucosa and skin of the lower lip.

The *lingual nerve* is the final branch of the posterior division of the mandibular nerve. It lies between the tensor palati and lateral pterygoid muscles and is joined by the chorda tympani branch of the facial nerve. The nerve passes downwards and forwards between the mandibular ramus and the medial pterygoid muscle, being here anterior to and at a slightly deeper level than the inferior alveolar nerve. After passing inferiorly to the origin from the mandible of the superior constrictor muscle of the pharynx it runs, covered only by the buccal mucosa, on the deep aspect of the mandible medial to the roots of the last molar tooth: it can here be palpated from inside the mouth. It leaves the gum, passing over the styloglossus, hyoglossus and genioglossus muscles and deep to the mylohyoid muscle. It here lies superior to the deep part of the sub-mandibular salivary gland and its duct (of Wharton), and suspended from it by two filaments is to be found the *submandibular ganglion*. The lingual nerve then divides into terminal branches which run just deep to the mucosa of the front of the tongue and of the floor of the mouth. The nerve is sensory to the presulcal tongue, the floor of the mouth and the mandibular gums: it also carries taste from the presulcal tongue.

THE SUBMANDIBULAR GANGLION AND ITS CONNECTIONS (Figs 36 and 48)

This ganglion is of the size of a pin head, and is of fusiform shape. It lies on the upper part of the hyoglossus muscle and is connected to the lingual nerve by two twigs. The ganglion receives a contribution from the nerve plexus around the facial artery and sends a branch to the submandibular salivary gland. It has motor, sympathetic and sensory roots.

The *motor root* is composed of preganglionic parasympathetic secretomotor fibres from the superior salivary nucleus via the facial nerve, its chorda tympani branch, the lingual nerve and finally the filament from the lingual nerve to the ganglion. The fibres synapse on the cells of the ganglion, whose axons form postganglionic parasympathetic secretomotor fibres which pass:

1 to the myoepithelium of the submandibular salivary gland via the twig from the ganglion to the gland, and
2 to the myoepithelium of the sublingual salivary gland, of the glands of the floor of the mouth and of the glands of the presulcal tongue via the filament which re-connects the ganglion with the lingual nerve.

The *sympathetic root* is composed of postganglionic sympathetic vasoconstrictor fibres from the superior cervical sympathetic ganglion via the plexus on the external carotid artery and the facial artery. The fibres pass through the ganglion without interruption to reach the sublingual and submandibular salivary glands, to the blood vessels of which they are vasomotor.

The *sensory root* comprises the proximal filament from the lingual nerve to the ganglion. The fibres from the mandibular division of the trigeminal nerve pass through the ganglion without interruption: they supply the mucosa of the submandibular and sublingual salivary glands and their ducts.

THE CENTRAL CONNECTIONS OF THE TRIGEMINAL NERVE These are discussed in Chapter 6

THE NUCLEAR CONNECTIONS OF THE TRIGEMINAL NERVE

General somatic afferent component (Figs 37 and 38)

Sensation is conveyed from the periphery to the trigeminal ganglion by the peripheral process (dendrite) of the pseudo-unipolar nerve cells of the ganglion: the sensation is conveyed to the central nervous system by

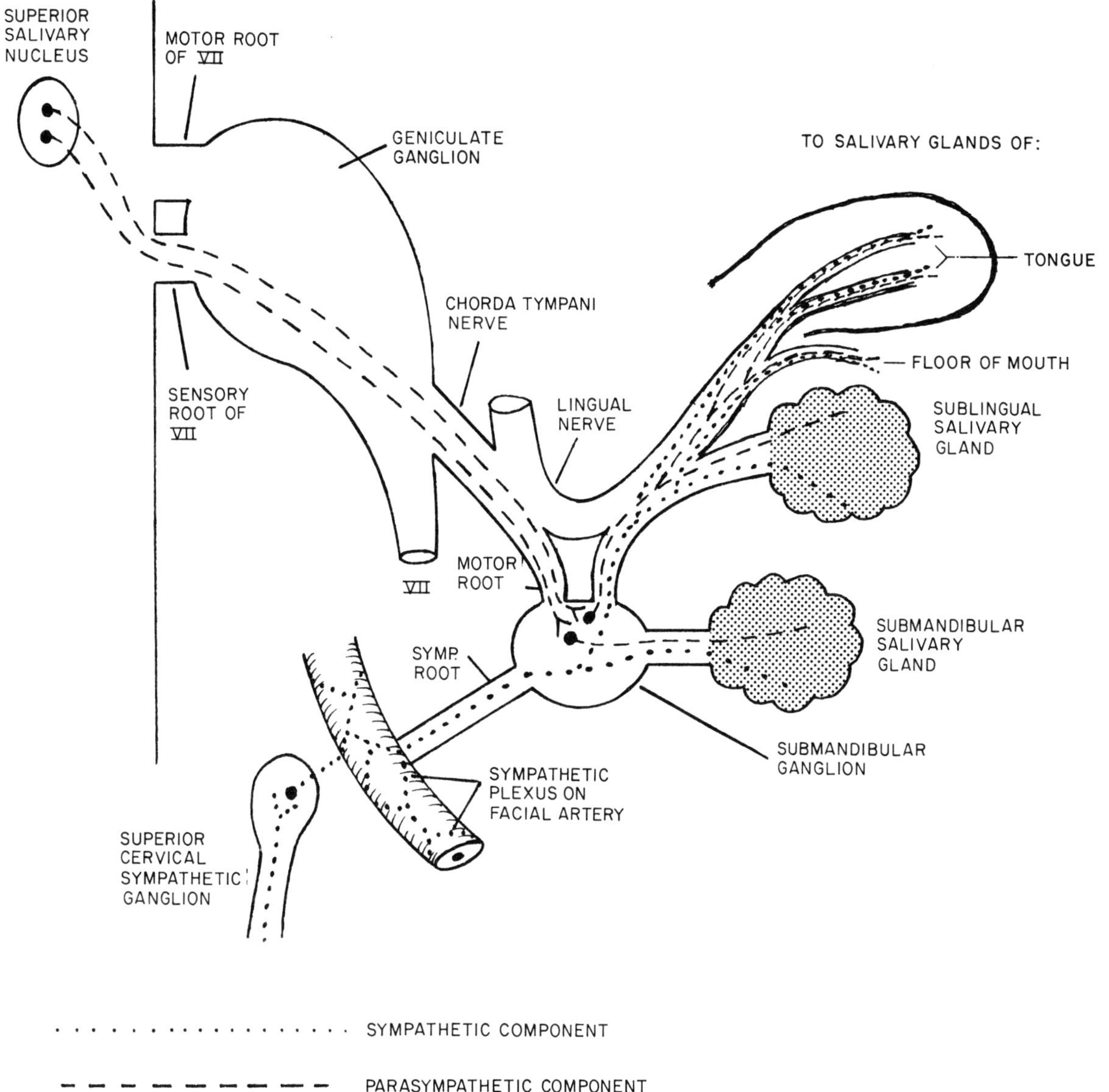

Fig 36 The connections of the submandibular ganglion.

the centrally-running process (axon) of the same cell. The sensation involved is cutaneous sensibility from the dermatome of the nerve — ie. scalp and face except for the angle of the jaw — plus sensation from the mucous membrane of cornea, conjunctiva, nasal cavity, mouth and presulcal tongue: the *pain and temperature fibres* from these regions terminate in the *nucleus of the spinal tract* of the trigeminal nerve: the representation of the three divisions of the nerve within the nucleus is however inverted. Thus fibres from the ophthalmic

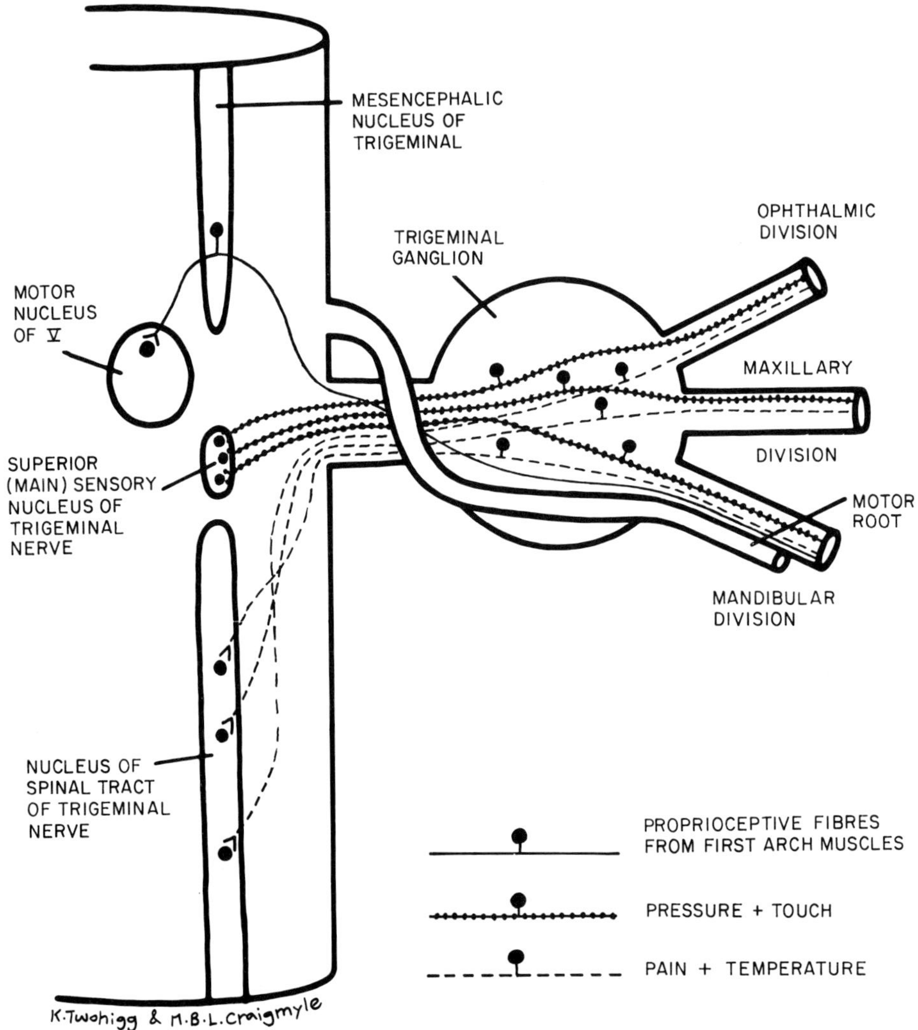

Fig 37   The sensory (GSA) component of the trigeminal nerve.

nerve pass to the lower end and fibres from the mandibular nerve end in the upper part of the nucleus. The maxillary nerve fibres pass to the middle of the nucleus.

Pressure and touch fibres from all three divisions of the trigeminal nerve pass to the *superior (main) sensory nucleus* of the trigeminal nerve. Efferents from the multipolar neurones of both nuclei (ie. superior sensory and of spinal tract) pass in the trigeminothalamic tract to the ventral posteromedial nucleus of the thalamus of the opposite side. The cell bodies of the third-order neurones in this nucleus send their axons via the internal capsule and the corona radiata to the postcentral gyrus of the cerebral cortex (Fig 7).

Proprioceptive fibres from the (first branchial arch) skeletal muscles innervated by the mandibular nerve *belong properly to the special visceral afferent group, but are conventionally dealt with under the general somatic afferent heading and this will be followed here.*

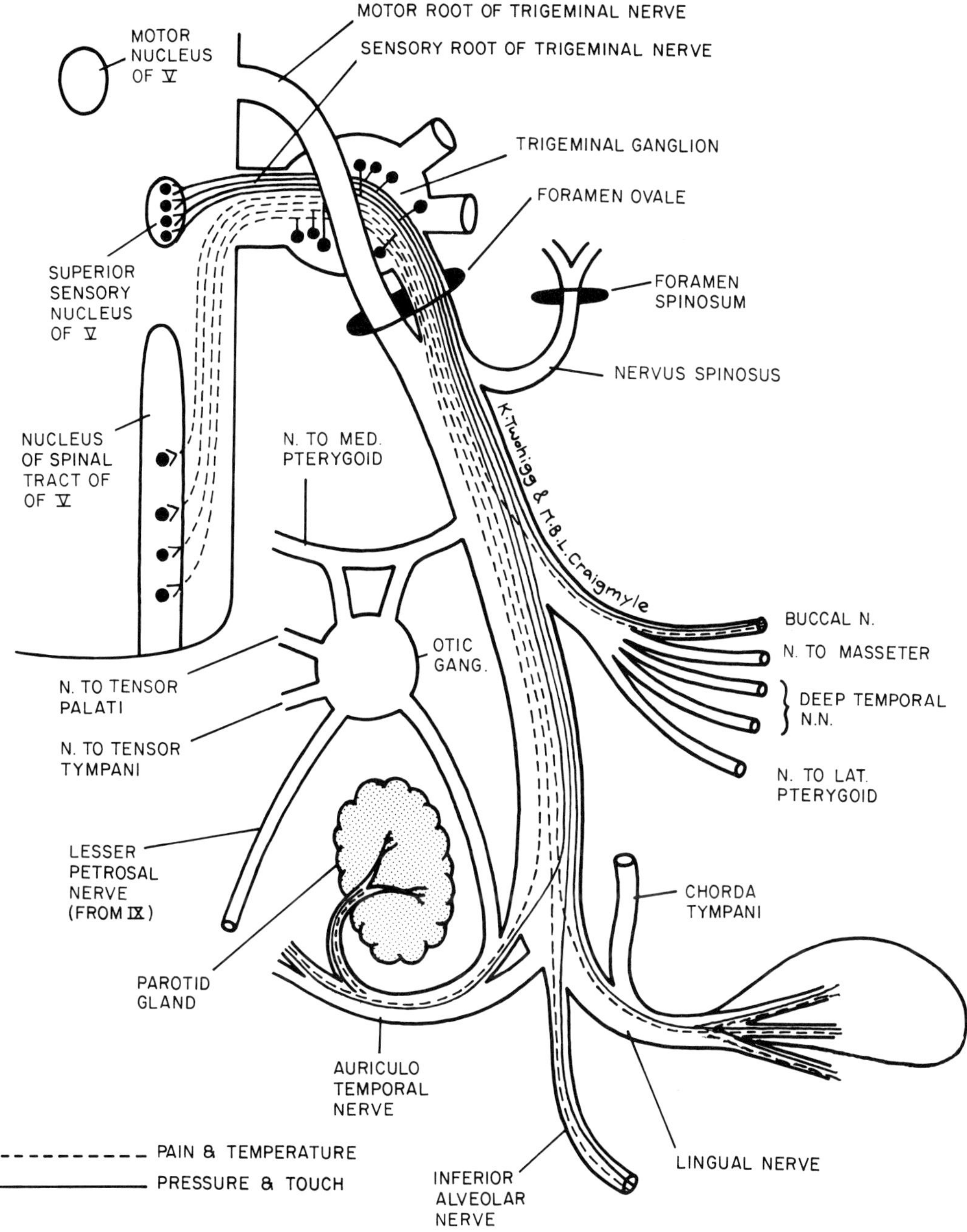

Fig 38 The distribution of the manibular division of the trigeminal nerve: the general somatic afferent component.

The fibres from the muscles are the dendritic processes of the pseudo-unipolar nerve cells in the mesencephalic nucleus of the trigeminal nerve, which lies in the midbrain. They enter the brain stem in the sensory root of the nerve, having passed through the ganglion without interruption and form, as they ascend, the mesencephalic tract of the trigeminal nerve. The axons of the nerve cells in the mesencephalic nucleus pass to the motor nucleus of the trigeminal nerve and relay on the neurones there. (Proprioceptive fibres from the extrinsic ocular muscles, from the muscles of facial expression and from the teeth also terminate in all probability in the mesencephalic nucleus of the trigeminal nerve.)

Special visceral (branchial) efferent component
(Figs 39 and 40)

The axons from the multipolar lower motor neurones located in the *motor nucleus of the trigeminal nerve* leave the brain stem in the motor root of the trigeminal nerve and pass into the mandibular nerve. They pass in the branches of the nerve to supply the skeletal muscles

derived from the mesoderm of the first branchial arch: temporalis, masseter, lateral pterygoid, medial pterygoid, mylohyoid, anterior belly of digastric, tensor tympani and tensor palati. The mandibular nerve is the nerve of the first branchial arch.

The nuclear connections of the trigeminal nerve are summarised in Figure 41.

LESIONS OF THE TRIGEMINAL NERVE

A complete lesion of the nerve results in anaesthesia, of the affected side, of:

1　the scalp anterior to the lambdoid suture
2　the face except the angle of the jaw
3　the cornea and conjunctiva
4　the mucosa of the nasal cavity
5　the mucosa of the mouth
6　the mucosa of the anterior two-thirds of the tongue. Loss of taste can also occur here if the chorda tympani component is lost.

In addition, the loss of masticatory muscles causes the mandible to be thrust to the affected side when the mouth is opened.

The trigeminal nerve subserves the afferent side of the following reflexes:

1　corneal (lids close when cornea touched)
2　lacrimal (lacrimation on corneal irritation)
3　chewing (salivation when food is in the mouth)
4　sneezing (when nasal mucosa is irritated)

A lesion of one of the divisions of the nerve will lead to anaesthesia in the skin and mucosa supplied by that division and additionally to motor loss if the division affected is the mandibular. Referred pain from one division of the nerve to another is common, e.g.:

eating very cold foods can cause earache.
dental caries can cause earache.

Trigeminal neuralgia (tic douloureux) can be a very intractible condition in some patients. The aetiology is obscure. Complete division of the sensory root of the nerve will effect a cure at the expense of a neuropathic keratitis due to the loss of the corneal reflex. The sensory root can, however, be divided in such fashion as to leave the ophthalmic fibres (which lie in the superomedial part

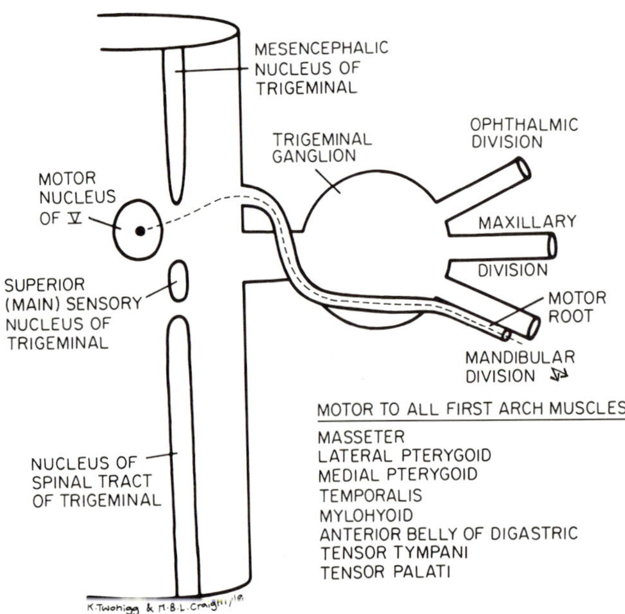

Fig 39　The motor (SVE) component of the trigeminal nerve.

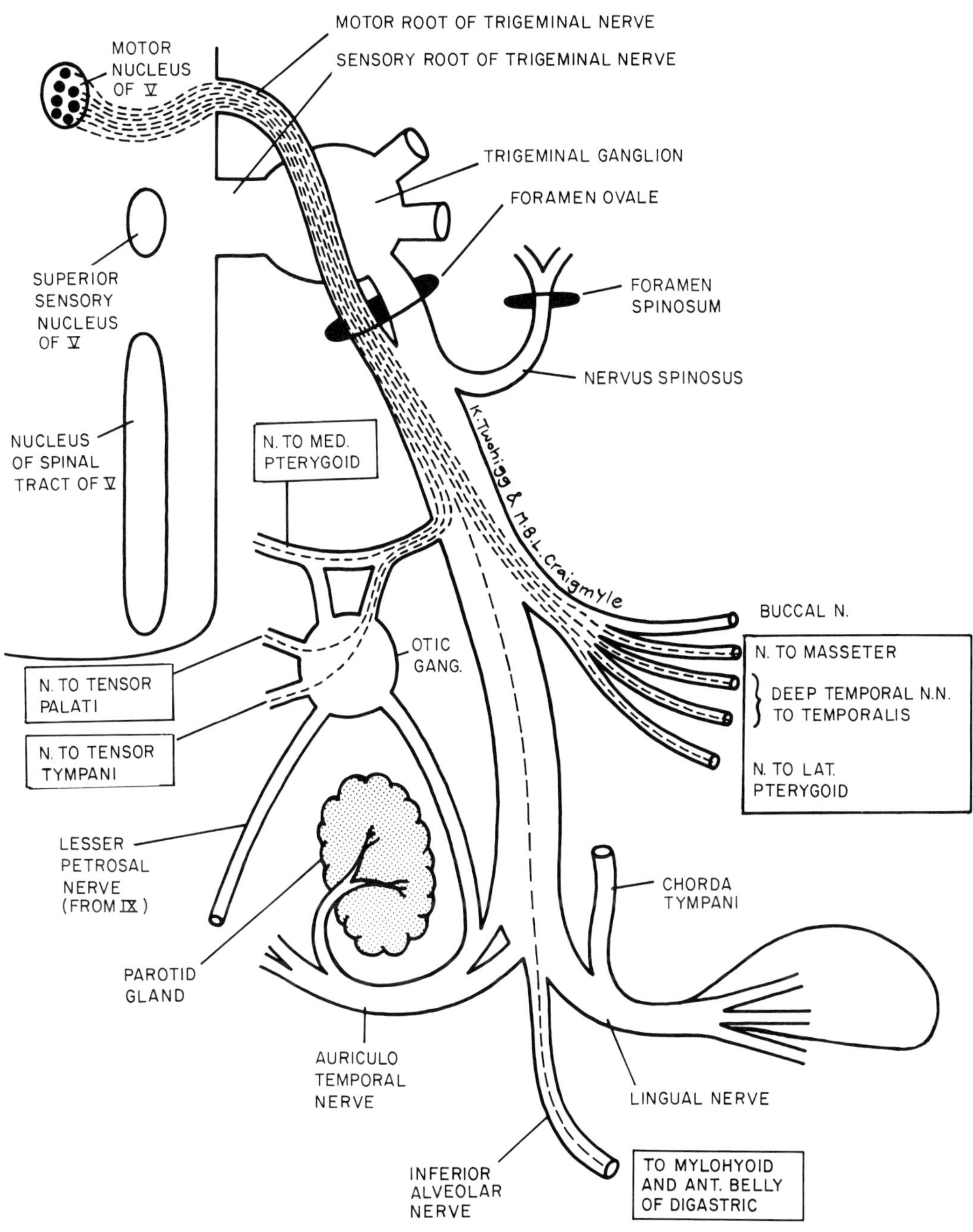

Fig 40 The distribution of the mandibular division of the trigeminal nerve: the special visceral (branchial) efferent component.

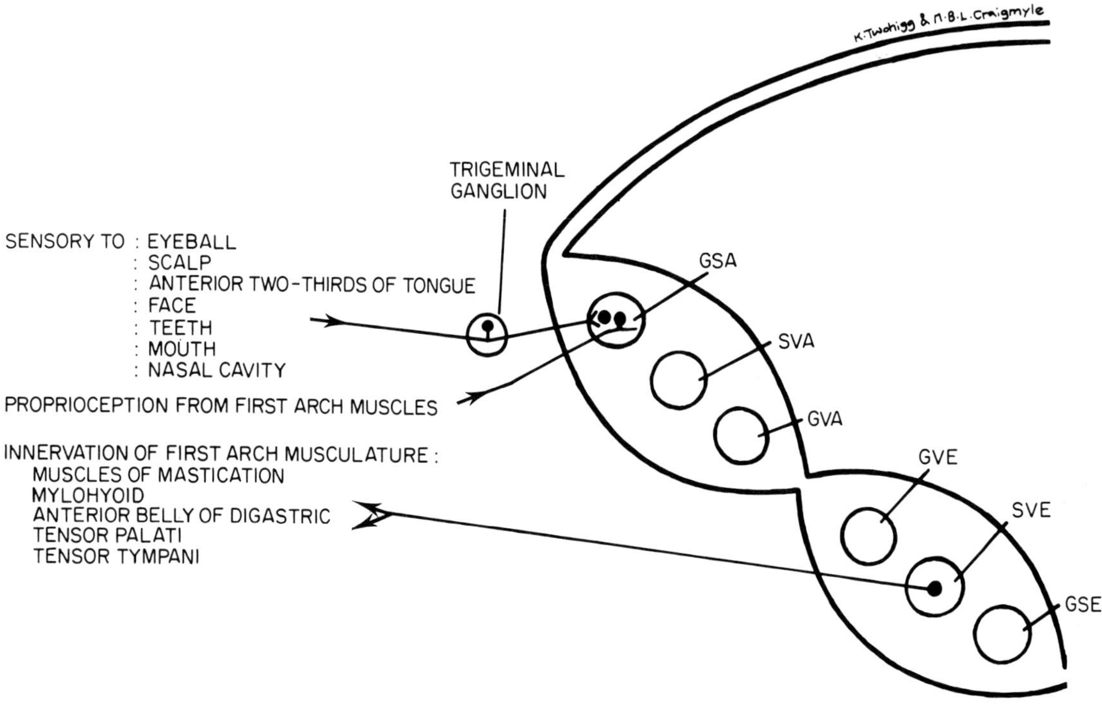

Fig 41   Summary of the nuclear connections of the trigeminal nerve.

of the root) intact in cases of maxillary or mandibular nerve neuralgia. In neuralgia of the ophthalmic division, the best cure is obtained by dividing the spinal tract of the nerve where it lies superficially between the lower part of the olive and the cuneate tract: tactile sensations are not interrupted by such a manoeuvre and so the corneal reflex is retained.

Because of the central dissociation of the afferent fibres within the brain stem, central lesions of the nerve can sometimes result in interference with one sensory modality alone. A lesion in the pons affecting only the superior sensory nucleus can result in loss of touch sensations over the trigeminal area, but pain and temperature sensations are not disrupted. Conversely, a lesion of the nucleus of the spinal tract of the trigeminal nerve in the medulla results in anaesthesia and thermal loss: it is to be remembered in this connection that the mandibular nerve afferents terminate in the upper part of the spinal nucleus and the ophthalmic afferents in the lowest.

SITES OF LESION

1 *In the brain stem*

   (a)   Tumours
   (b)   Vascular lesions
   (c)   Syringobulbia
   (d)   Thrombosis of the posterior inferior cerebellar artery

2 *Between the pons and trigeminal ganglion*

   (a)   Tumours
   (b)   Aneurysms
   (c)   Syphilitic meningitis

3 *In the trigeminal ganglion*

   (a)   Tumours of the ganglion
   (b)   Hypophyseal tumours
   (c)   Meningiomata or other tumours
   (d)   Mastoiditis spreading to the inferior petrosal sinus (Gradenigo's syndrome)
   (e)   Herpes zoster of the ganglion

10

THE ABDUCENT NERVE

ORIGIN, COURSE AND DISTRIBUTION (Fig 42)

This nerve arises from the groove between the caudal end of the pons and the cranial end of the pyramid of the medulla oblongata (Fig 19). It enters the pontine cistern and runs forward and upwards on the clivus of the occipital bone. After piercing the dura mater it passes medial to the apex of the petrous portion of the temporal bone and runs along the lateral wall of the cavernous sinus below the ophthalmic division and above the maxillary division of the trigeminal nerve. It usually communicates with the first of these. The nerve enters the orbit through the superior orbital fissure and passes through the common tendinous ring of origin of the rectus muscles. It enters the orbital surface of the lateral rectus muscle (Fig 42).

CENTRAL CONNECTIONS OF THE ABDUCENT NERVE See Chapter 6

NUCLEAR CONNECTIONS OF THE ABDUCENT NERVE

General somatic efferent component: *the abducent nucleus* (Fig 43)

This nucleus lies in the pontine part of the floor of the fourth ventricle, into which it bulges. The swelling is known as the facial colliculus because the abducent nucleus is overlaid by a layer of nerve fibres belonging to the facial nerve. The fibres from the lower motor neurones in the nucleus supply the lateral rectus muscle.

General somatic afferent component: *the mesencephalic nucleus of the trigeminal nerve* (Fig 44)

The proprioceptive fibres from the lateral rectus muscle terminate in the mesencephalic nucleus of the trigeminal nerve: whether they reach the brain stem in the abducent nerve or in the sensory root of the trigeminal nerve is as yet unresolved.

The nuclear connections of the abducent nerve are summarised in Figure 45.

LESIONS OF THE ABDUCENT NERVE

The abducent nerve often becomes stretched in conditions in which the intracranial pressure is raised, because of its long intracranial course and the fact that in such conditions the brain stem is displaced caudally. There is medial squint (convergent strabismus) on the affected side, with resultant diplopia.

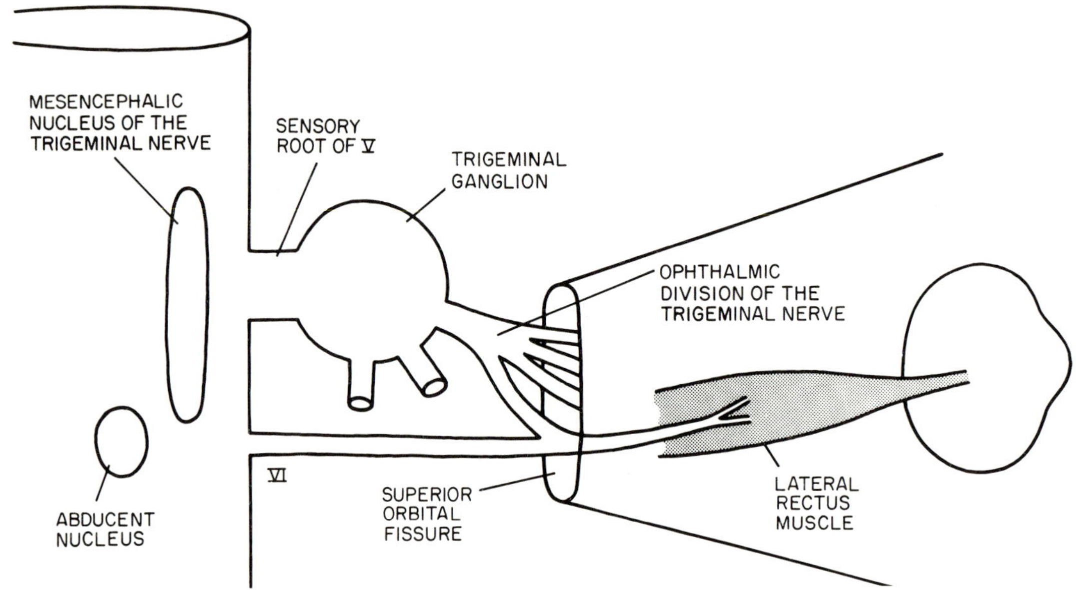

Fig 42   The distribution of the abducent nerve.

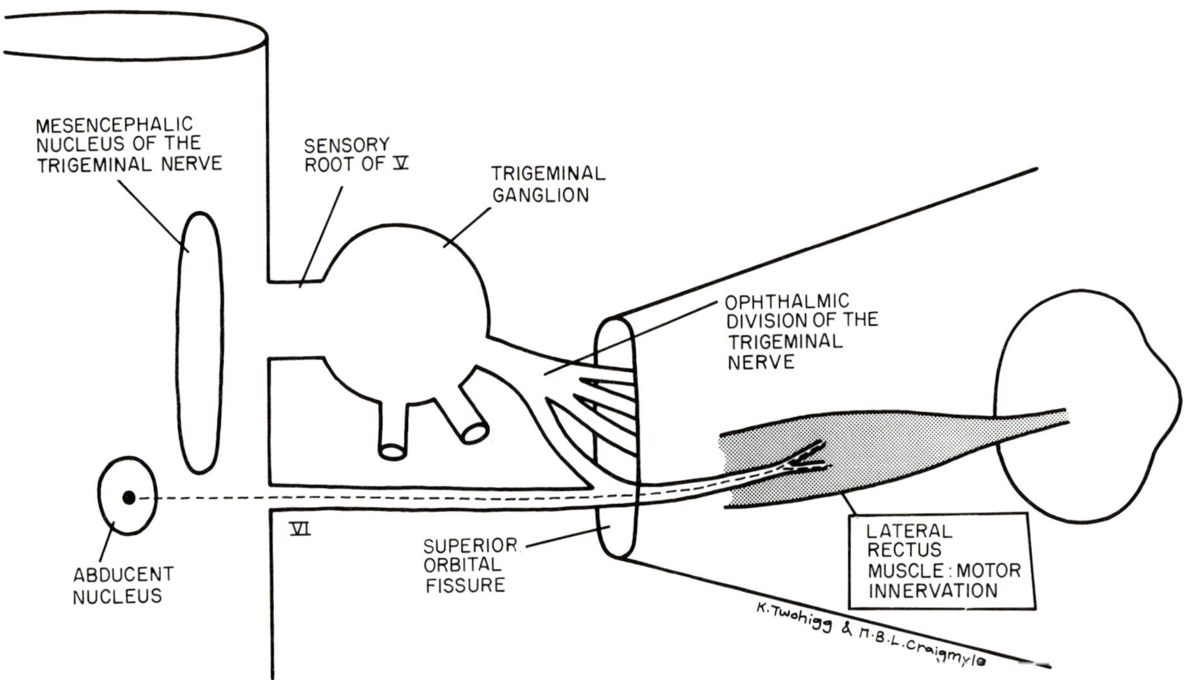

Fig 43   The distribution of the abducent nerve: the general somatic efferent component.

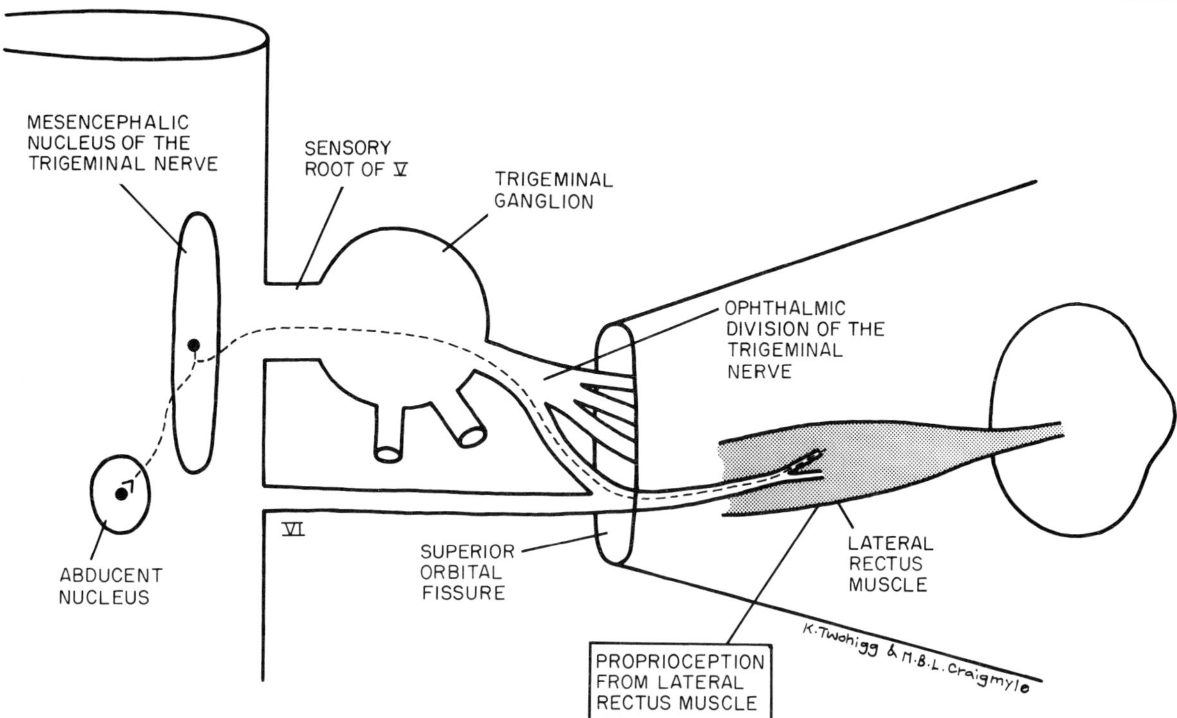

Fig 44   The distribution of the abducent nerve: the general somatic afferent component.

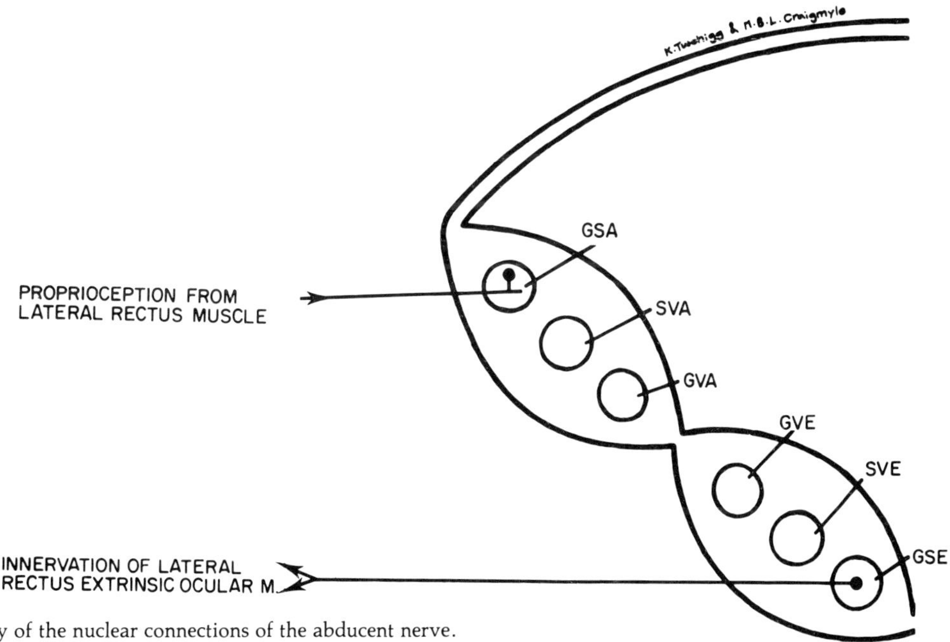

Fig 45   Summary of the nuclear connections of the abducent nerve.

SITES OF LESION

1 *In the brain stem*

(a) Poliomyelitis
(b) Multiple sclerosis
(c) Gliomata
(d) Vascular lesions
(e) Wernick's encephalopathy

2 *In the basilar area*

(a) Aneurysm of the basilar artery
(b) Basal meningitis
(c) Neoplasia of nasopharynx or paranasal air sinuses
(d) Sarcoid
(e) Herpes zoster
(f) Fractures

3 *At the petrous tip*

(a) Inflammation of the petrous temporal bone and thrombosis of the superior petrosal sinus secondary to middle ear infection or mastoiditis.

(b) Lateral sinus thrombosis resultant from mastoiditis, or a posterior cranial fossa abscess can cause raised intracranial pressure and sixth nerve stretching.

4 *In the area of the cavernous sinus*

(a) Cavernous sinus thrombosis
(b) Intrasellar tumours
(c) Aneurysm of the internal carotid artery
(d) Aneurysm of the posterior communicating artery
(e) Temporal lobe displacement or enlargement, causing the nerve to be stretched over the tentorum cerebelli.

5 *In the orbit*

(a) Retro-orbital tumours: meningiomata
                          gliomata
                          haemangiomata
                          carcinomata

11

THE FACIAL NERVE

ORIGIN, COURSE AND DISTRIBUTION (Fig 46)

The nerve arises by two roots, larger motor and smaller sensory, from the pons in the interval between the olive and the inferior cerebellar peduncle (Fig 19). (The sensory root is often called the nervus intermedius because it lies between the (large) motor root of the facial and the vestibulocochlear nerve.) Both roots enter the internal acoustic meatus and unite to form a single nerve which then enters the facial canal of the temporal bone. In the canal it crosses above the vestibule of the inner ear to reach the medial wall of the epitypanic recess of the middle ear: here is exhibits a gangliform swelling (geniculate ganglion) and bends backwards to run along the medial wall of the middle ear above the promontory. The greater petrosal nerve is given off via the geniculate ganglion. The facial nerve bends inferiorly to pass medial to the aditus to the tympanic antrum which lies in the posterior wall of the tympanic cavity to emerge from the base of the skull at the stylomastoid foramen. Before emerging, it gives off the nerve to stapedius, the chorda tympani nerve, and a communicating branch to the auricular branch of the vagus. Immediately on emerging from the stylomastoid foramen the facial nerve gives off the posterior auricular nerve. The facial nerve then passes between the styloid process and the posterior belly of the digastric muscle, giving a branch to the latter in passing. The facial nerve next gives a branch to the stylohyoid muscle before entering the parotid gland on its posteromedial aspect. Within the gland substance the nerve divides into five sets of terminal branches, temporal, zygomatic, buccal, marginal mandibular and cervical. The temporal and cervical branches emerge respectively from the superior and inferior aspects of the parotid gland and the other three sets from the front of the gland.

SUMMARY OF BRANCHES OF THE FACIAL NERVE

1   Within the facial canal

    (a)   the greater petrosal nerve
    (b)   the nerve to stapedius
    (c)   the chorda tympani nerve

2   In the neck

    (a)   the posterior auricular nerve
    (b)   the nerve to the posterior belly of the digastric muscle
    (c)   the nerve to stylohyoid

55

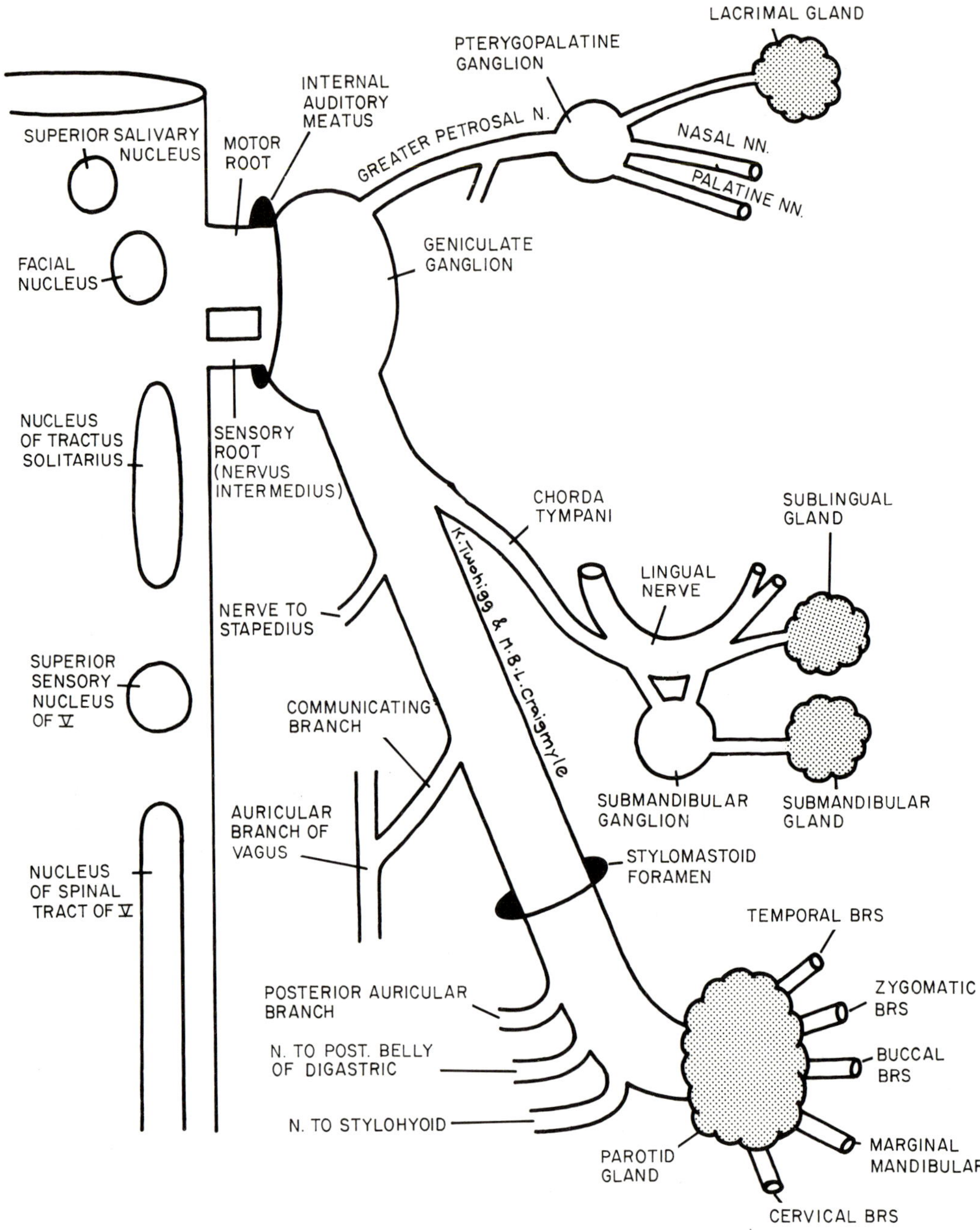

Fig 46   The distribution of the facial nerve.

3   On the face

  (a)   temporal
  (b)   zygomatic
  (c)   buccal
  (d)   marginal mandibular
  (e)   cervical

The greater petrosal nerve

This nerve reaches the middle cranial fossa by issuing from the facial canal through a tiny foramen on the anterior surface of the petrous portion of the temporal bone. It runs forwards, passing under the trigeminal ganglion and over the foramen lacerum to unite with the deep petrosal nerve, a branch from the sympathetic plexus on the internal carotid artery. The nerve so formed enters the pterygoid canal as the nerve of that canal to reach the pterygopalatine fossa and terminate in the pterygopalatine ganglion.

The nerve to the stapedius muscle

This twig is given off by the facial nerve as it runs down in the facial canal in the posteromedial corner of the middle ear cavity.

The chorda tympani nerve

This branch is given off by the facial nerve 5 mm above its exit from the stylomastoid foramen. The nerve runs upwards and forwards in a bony canal and enters the tympanic cavity via a minute foramen on its posterior wall. It passes forwards in the mucosa on the inner aspect of the tympanic membrane, crossing medial to the neck of the malleus, before leaving the tympanic cavity via a small bony canal in its anterior wall. This canal opens into the infratemporal fossa via the squamotympanic fissure of the tympanic bone. The chorda tympani nerve then passes medial to the spine of the sphenoid bone, often grooving it, before passing between the tensor palati and the lateral pterygoid muscles. It is crossed by the middle meningeal artery, the two roots of the auriculotemporal nerve and the inferior alveolar nerve before ending by joining the lingual nerve.

The communicating branch to the auricular branch of the vagus

This twig is given off by the facial nerve in the facial canal and joins the auricular branch of the vagus which is running in a canal in the temporal bone (mastoid canaliculus) which is cutting across the facial canal. The nerve so formed is distributed to the skin of the cranial surface of the pinna of the ear and of the postero-inferior wall of the external auditory meatus.

The posterior auricular nerve

This branch of the facial nerve is given off after the parent nerve emerges from the stylomastoid foramen. It passes upwards between the mastoid process and the external auditory meatus before dividing into an auricular branch distributed to the muscles of the pinna and the auricularis posterior muscle, and a larger occipital branch which follows the superior nuchal line of the occipital bone to reach the occipital belly of the occipitofrontalis muscle.

The nerve to the posterior belly of the digastric muscle

This small twig is given off as the facial nerve passes between the digastric muscle and the styloid process.

The nerve to the stylohyoid muscle

This small twig is given off by the facial nerve just before it enters the substance of the parotid gland.

The *temporal branches* arise from the facial nerve in the parotid gland and emerge from the upper pole of the gland. They cross the zygomatic arch to reach and supply:

  orbicularis oculi
  the frontal belly of occipitofrontalis
  auricularis anterior
  auricularis superior
  the intrinsic muscles of the pinna

The *zygomatic branches* arise in the parotid gland and emerge to cross the zygomatic bone to supply orbicularis oculi and the zygomatic muscles.

The *buccal branches* arise in the substance of the parotid gland and after emerging from the front of the gland pass forwards horizontally to supply:

zygomaticus minor
zygomaticus major
levator labii superioris
levator anguli oris
levator labii superioris alaequae nasi
buccinator
orbicularis oris
the small muscles of the nose

The marginal mandibular branch

This arises in the parotid gland substance and emerges to run forwards below the angle and the posterior part of the body of the mandible deep to the platysma muscle. It supplies:

risorius
platysma
depressor anguli oris
the muscles of lower lip
the muscles of chin

The *cervical branch* issues from the lower pole of the parotid gland to reach and supply the platysma muscle.

CENTRAL CONNECTIONS OF THE FACIAL NERVE

See Chapter 6.

NUCLEAR CONNECTIONS OF THE FACIAL NERVE

Special visceral (branchial) efferent component: *the facial nucleus* (Fig 47)

Fully three-quarters of the fibres in the facial nerve are of this type. They arise in the facial nucleus in the pons and leave the brain stem in the motor root of the nerve. The facial nucleus lies in the ventrolateral part of the reticular formation of the pons, and the fibres from the lower motor neurones in the nucleus pass dorsomedially towards the floor of the fourth ventricle before passing around the abducent nucleus and then between the nucleus of the spinal tract of the trigeminal nerve and the facial nucleus to regain the reticular formation before emerging from the pons: this unusual course is indicative of the fact that the facial nucleus underwent migration during development. The fibres are distributed to:

the stapedius muscle
the posterior belly of the digastric muscle
the stylohyoid muscle
all the muscles of facial expression

Since the facial nerve is the nerve of the second branchial arch, these muscles must be derived from the mesoderm of that arch.

General visceral efferent component: *the superior salivary nucleus* (Fig 48)

Preganglionic parasympathetic fibres pass from the superior salivary nucleus into the facial nerve via its motor root. They are distributed:

1   Through the greater petrosal nerve to the pterygopalatine ganglion where they synapse: the postganglionic fibres pass via the zygomatic nerve and its communicating branch to the lacrimal nerve to the myoepithelium of the lacrimal gland and via the nasal and palatine branches of the ganglion to the myoepithelium of the salivary glands of the nose and palate.

2   Through the chorda tympani nerve to the lingual nerve and so to the submandibular ganglion where they relay: postganglionic fibres then pass back into the lingual nerve to reach the myoepithelium of the submandibular and sublingual glands and of the salivary glands in the floor of the mouth and the tongue.

Special visceral afferent component: *the nucleus of the tractus solitarius* (Fig 49)

Taste fibres from the tongue anterior to the sulcus terminalis pass in the lingual nerve to the chorda tympani branch of the facial nerve. The (pseudo-unipolar) cell bodies lie in the geniculate ganglion and their efferents enter the brain stem in the nervus intermedius to terminate in the upper part of the nucleus of the tractus solitarius. Similarly, taste fibres from the palate pass in the greater and lesser palatine nerves to the pterygopalatine ganglion (through which they pass without interruption) and thence to the facial nerve via the nerve of the pterygoid canal and the greater petrosal nerve.

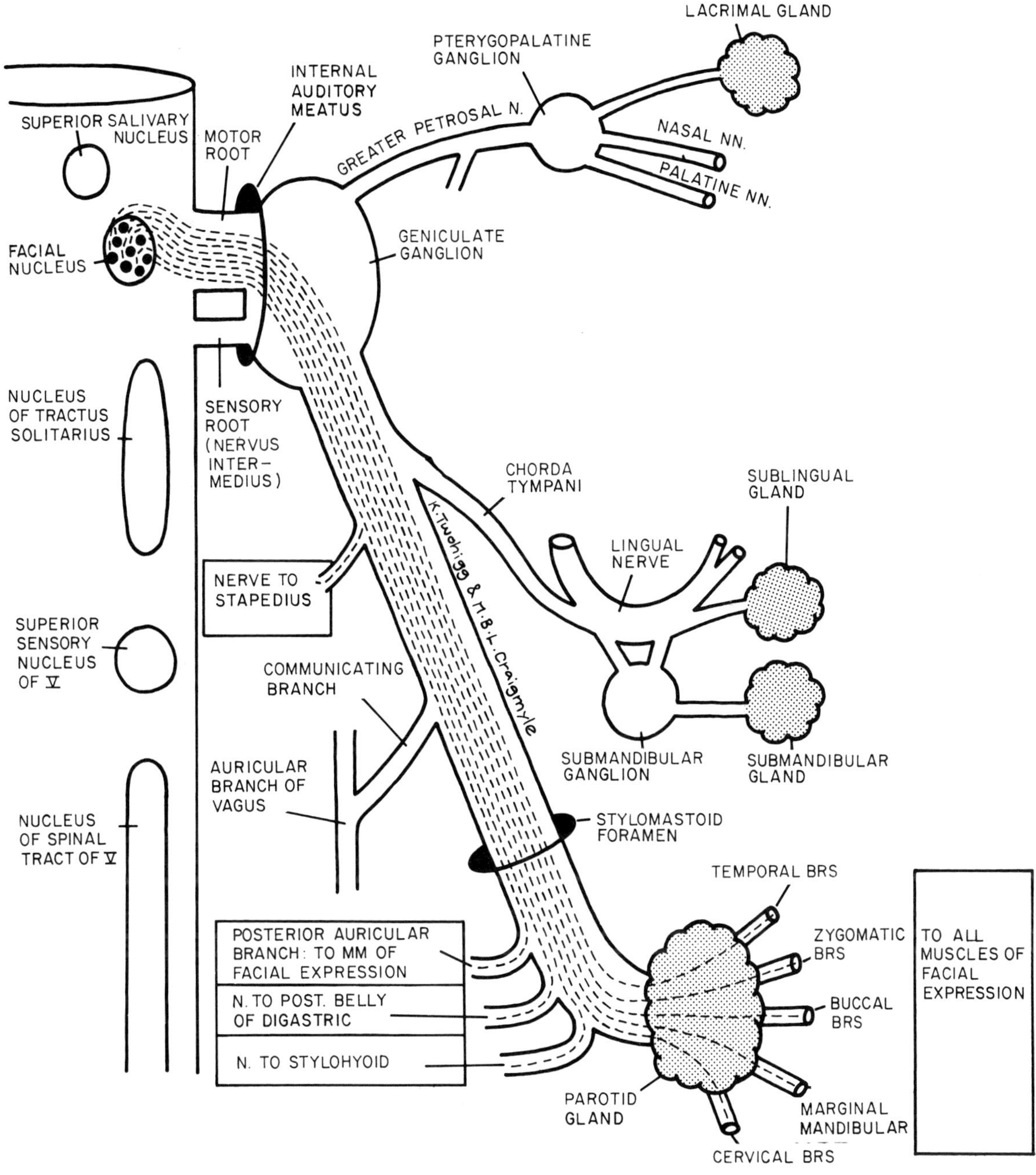

Fig 47 The distribution of the facial nerve: the special visceral (branchial) efferent component.

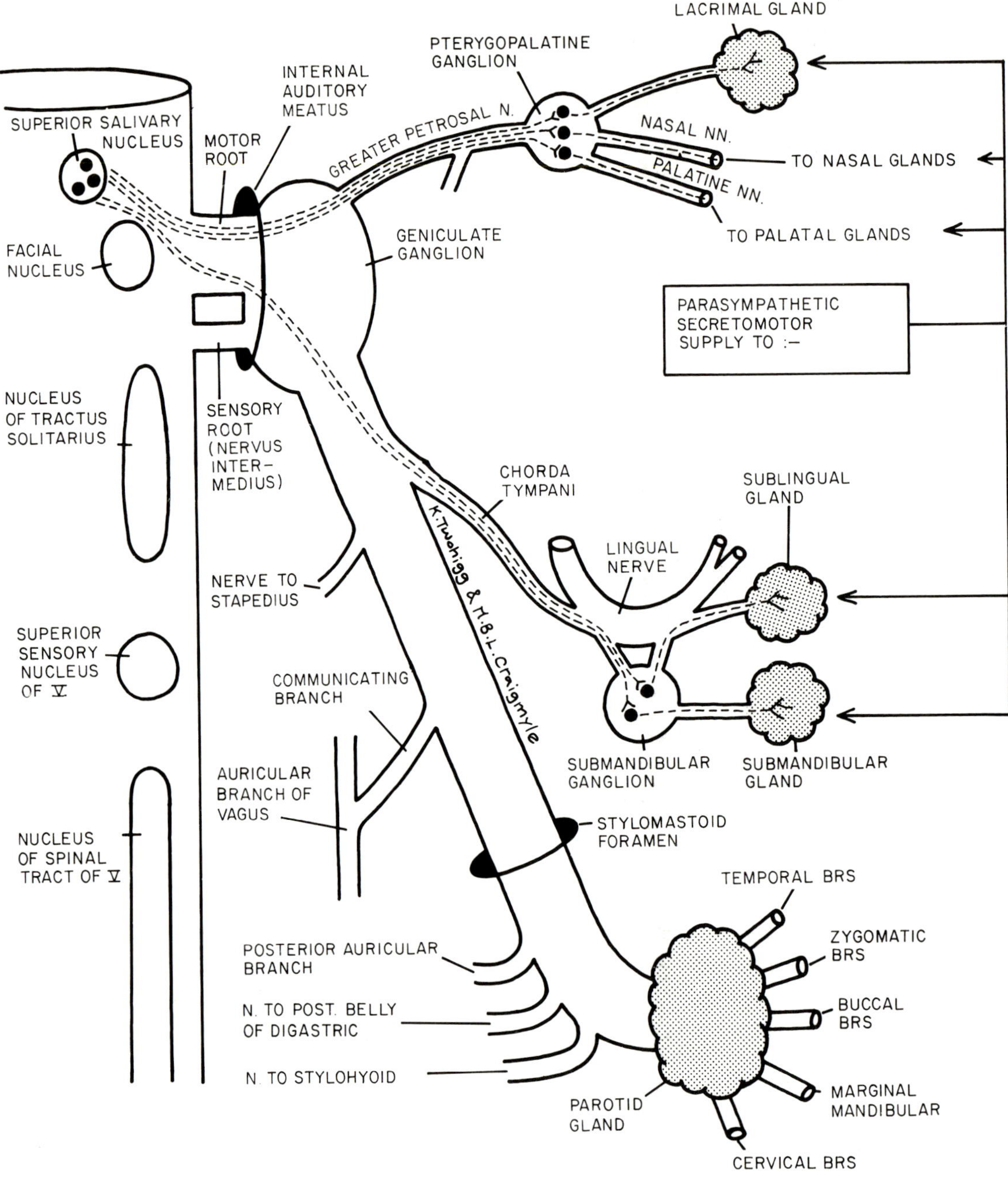

Fig 48 The distribution of the facial nerve: the general visceral efferent component.

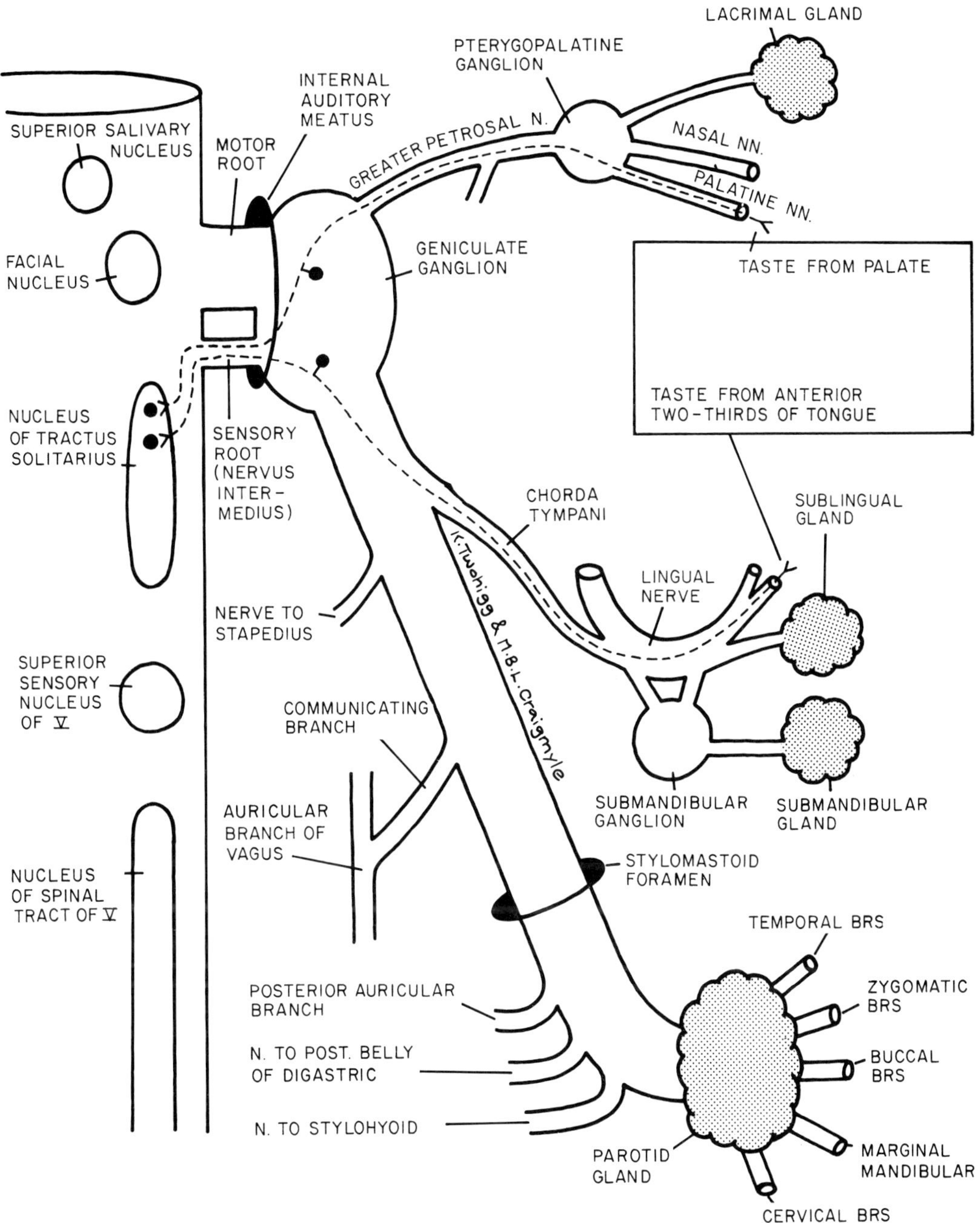

Fig 49 The distribution of the facial nerve: the special visceral afferent (taste) component.

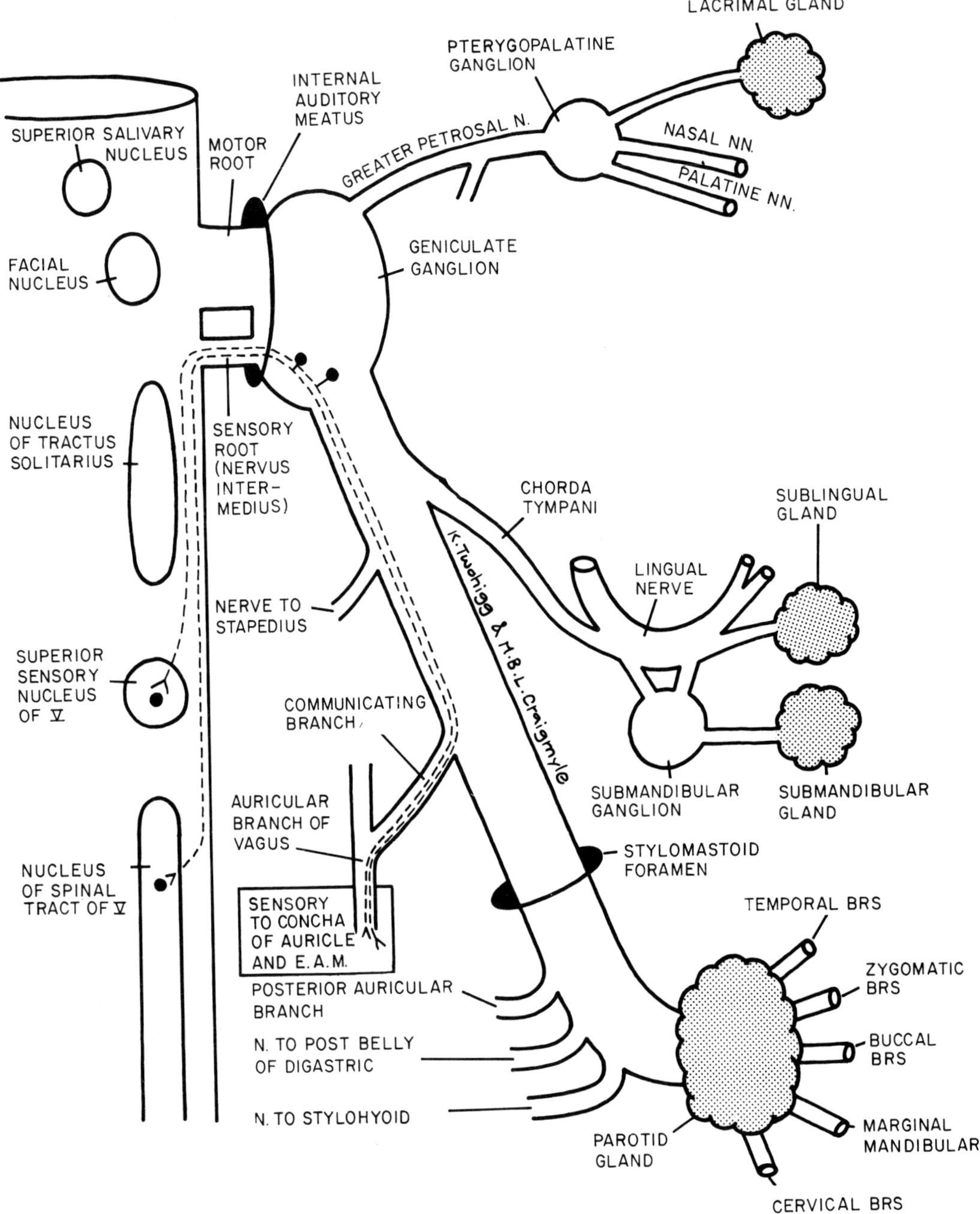

Fig 50   The distribution of the facial nerve: general somatic afferent component.

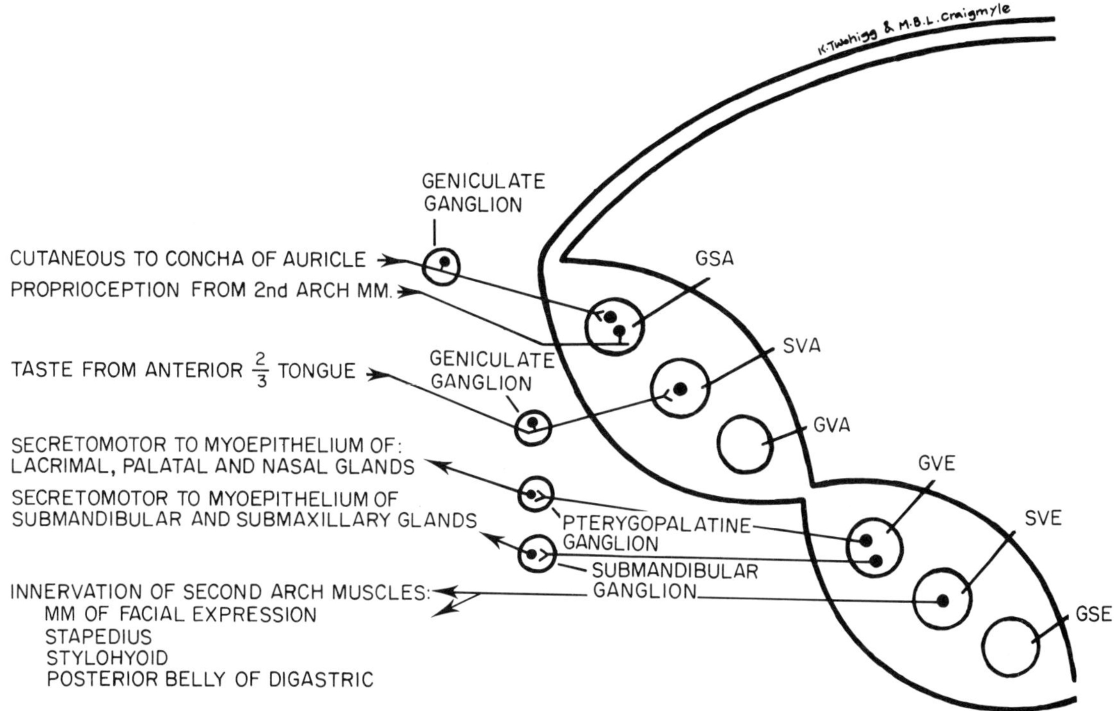

Fig 51 Summary of the nuclear connections of the facial nerve.

General somatic afferent component: *the trigeminal nuclei* (Fig 50)

Pseudo-unipolar nerve cells in the geniculate ganglion receive cutaneous sensibility from the pinna and the external acoustic meatus via the auricular branch of the vagus and its communicating branch with the facial nerve. The centrally-directed process will terminate either on the superior sensory nucleus of the trigeminal nerve (tactile sensation) or in the nucleus of the spinal tract of the trigeminal nerve (painful and thermal sensibility).

The nuclear connections of the facial nerve are summarised in Figure 51.

LESIONS OF THE FACIAL NERVE

The clinical picture presented by a lesion of the facial nerve will depend on whether the upper or the lower motor neurone is affected. In both instances there will be unilateral facial paralysis. In the case of an upper motor neurone lesion, the lower half of the face will be more severely affected than the upper because the cerebral hemisphere has a greater influence on the lower part of the face on the opposite side. In the instance of a lower motor neurone lesion, all the facial muscles on the same side are affected. The commonest cause of lower motor neurone damage of the facial nerve is Bell's palsy in which the nerve is inflamed in the facial canal. Loss of tone in the orbicularis oculi muscle allows the lids (and therefore the puncta lacrimalia) to flop forward so that tears run down the face on the affected side. Loss of buccinator tone allows food to collect in the cheek. Loss of function in orbicularis oris permits saliva to dribble from the corner of the mouth on the affected side. Involvement of the chorda tympani in Bell's palsy means also that there is taste loss on the front of the tongue on the affected side. Facial paralysis in the absence of such taste loss means that the facial nerve has been damaged distal to the point where it is joined by the chorda tympani.

SITES OF LESION

1 *Supranuclear lesion of upper motor neurone*
Cerebral cardiovascular accident

2 *Within the pons*

   (a) Vascular lesion within the brain stem
   (b) Poliomyelitis
   (c) Multiple sclerosis
   (d) Brain-stem glioma
   (e) Wernick's encephalopathy

3 *At the cerebellopontine angle*

   (a) Meningiomata
   (b) Haemangioblastomata
   (c) Tumours of VIII nerve

   (d) Cholesteatomata
   (e) Cerebellar tumours
   (f) Aneurysm of the basilar artery

4 *Within the temporal bone*

   (a) Fractures of skull
   (b) Middle ear infections
   (c) Mastoid infections
   (d) Herpes zoster
   (e) Epidermoid within the temporal bone
   (f) Inflammation of the nerve

5 *In the neck and face*

   (a) Lymphadenitis of deep cervical nodes
   (b) Tumours of the parotid
   (c) Trauma

12

THE GLOSSOPHARYNGEAL NERVE

ORIGIN, COURSE AND DISTRIBUTION (Fig 52)

The glossopharyngeal nerve arises as several rootlets from the medulla oblongata at the cranial end of the groove between the olive and the inferior cerebellar penduncle (Fig 19). After crossing the jugular tubercle of the occipital bone it leaves the skull via the jugular foramen accompanied by the vagus and accessory nerves and the inferior petrosal and sigmoid sinuses. Within or just below the foramen the nerve exhibits a small inconstant superior ganglion which gives off no branches, and a larger inferior ganglion, which gives off a tympanic branch and a communicating branch to the auricular branch of the vagus nerve.

The glossopharyngeal nerve descends between the internal jugular vein and the internal carotid artery, passing with them and the vagus, accessory and hypoglossal nerves deep to the styloid process and the muscles arising from it. The nerve gives off a carotid branch and then curves round the stylopharyngeus muscle, supplying it as it does so. The glossopharyngeal nerve sends sensory branches to the pharyngeal plexus (which is completed by the cranial accessory and the vagus nerves) and to the tonsillar plexus (which is joined by the lesser palatine nerve). The glossopharyngeal

nerve crosses the triangular space between the superior and middle constrictors of the pharynx and the hyoglossus muscle and sends a twig of supply to the stylopharyngeus muscle, before terminating by sending two lingual branches to the mucosa of the posterior one-third of the tongue.

THE BRANCHES OF THE GLOSSOPHARYNGEAL NERVE

The tympanic branch

This is given off from the inferior ganglion. It passes into the tympanic canaliculus in the wall of the jugular foramen by which means it reaches the medial wall of the middle ear cavity. Here it breaks up on the surface of the promontory into the tympanic plexus which is joined by (caroticotympanic) branches from the sympathetic plexus on the internal carotid artery. From the plexus, branches are sent to the mucosa of the tympanic cavity, of the mastoid air cells and of the pharyngo-tympanic tube. The plexus also gives off:

The *lesser petrosal nerve*. This emerges from the anterior aspect of the petrous portion of the temporal

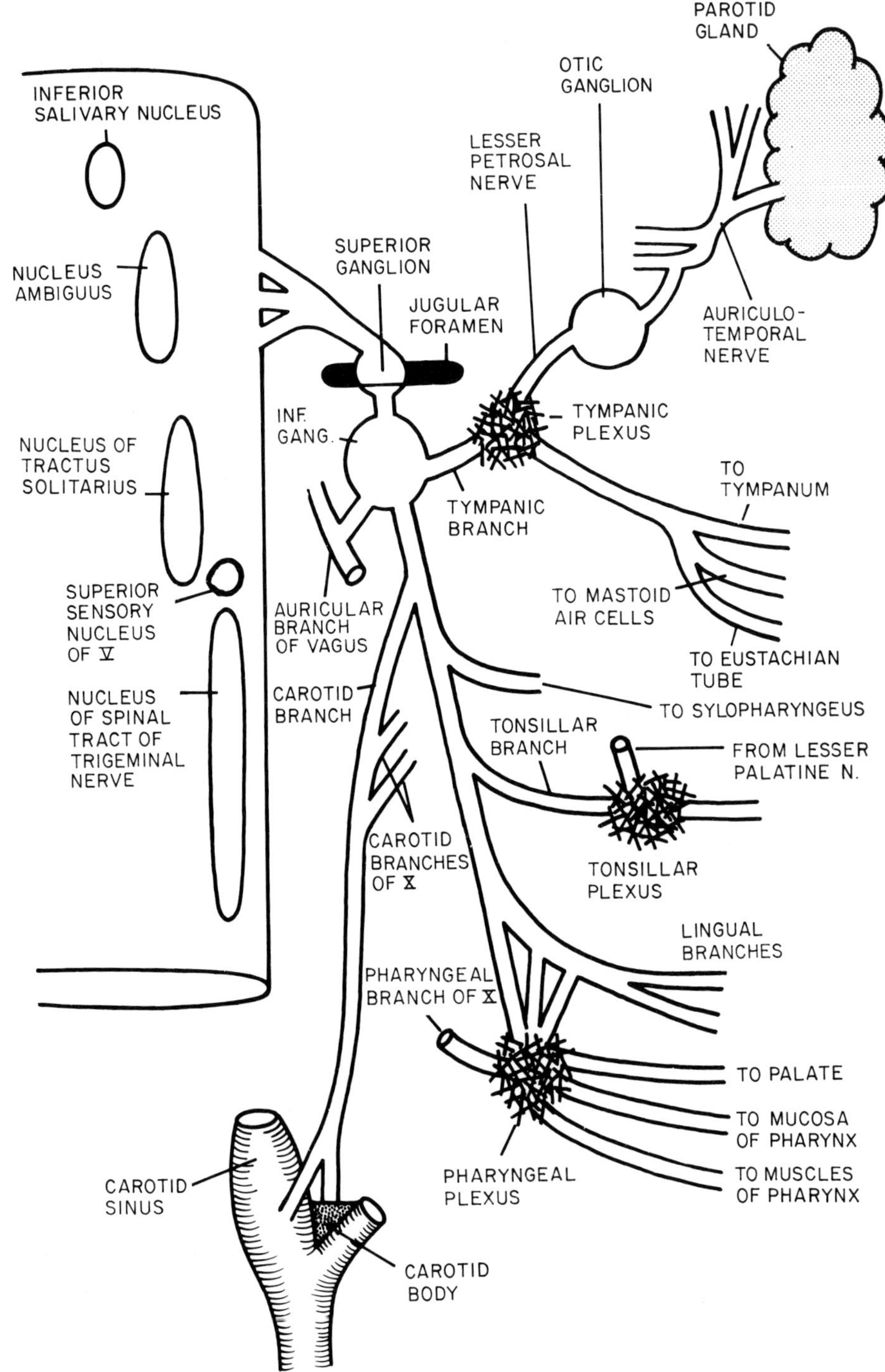

Fig 52   The distribution of the glossopharyngeal nerve.

bone through a small foramen lateral to the foramen for the greater petrosal nerve. The nerve then passes through the foramen ovale to join the otic ganglion.

The *branch to the auricular branch of the vagus* is also given off from the inferior glossopharyngeal ganglion, and carries cutaneous fibres.

The carotid nerve

This branch, often duplicated, arises from the glossopharyngeal nerve just below the jugular foramen. It descends on the surface of the internal carotid artery to be distributed to the carotid sinus and carotid body.

The *muscular branch*: this twig supplies the stylopharyngeus muscle.

The pharyngeal branches

These are three or four sensory filaments which form the plexus on the middle constrictor muscle of the pharynx with the pharyngeal branch of the vagus. From the plexus, branches pass to:

1 the palatal muscles (except tensor palati)
2 the pharyngeal muscles (except stylopharyngeus and the lower part of the inferior constrictor muscle)
3 the mucosa of the pharynx

The *tonsillar branches:* these small filaments form, with the lesser palatine nerve, a tonsillar plexus which supplies the mucosa of tonsil, soft palate, and the fauces.

The lingual branches

Of these there are two: one supplies the circumvallate papillae and the other the mucosa of the posterior one-third of the tongue.

CENTRAL CONNECTIONS OF THE GLOSSOPHARYNGEAL NERVE. See Chapter 6

NUCLEAR CONNECTIONS OF THE GLOSSOPHARYNGEAL NERVE

General visceral efferent component: *the inferior salivary nucleus* (Fig 53)

The axons of the cell bodies in this nucleus are pregang-

lionic parasympathetic secretomotor. They pass via the tympanic branch of the nerve, the tympanic plexus and the lesser petrosal nerve to the otic ganglion where they synapse. The postganglionic fibres pass to the auriculotemporal nerve by which they are conveyed to the parotid gland to innervate the myoepithelial cells.

Special visceral efferent component: *the nucleus ambiguus* (Fig 54)

The axons of the lower motor neurones in the upper part of the nucleus ambiguus pass in the branch of the nerve to the stylopharyngeus muscle. The glossopharyngeal nerve is the nerve of the third pharyngeal arch so stylopharyngeus is (the only muscle) of third arch origin. Proprioceptive fibres from the muscle are believed to end in the mesencephalic nucleus of the trigeminal nerve.

General visceral afferent component: *the nucleus of the tractus solitarius* (Fig 55)

The inferior ganglion of the nerve contains pseudounipolar nerve cells. Their peripheral processes receive general visceral afferent sensations from:

mucosa of tympanum
mucosa of mastoid air cells
mucosa of eustachian tube
mucosa of posterior one-third of tongue (for taste
  see below)
mucosa of tonsil
mucosa of pharynx
mucosa of soft palate
mucosa of faucal region
baroreceptors of carotid sinus
chemoreceptors of carotid body

The central processes of the pseudo-unipolar nerve cells terminate in the *lower* part of the nucleus of the tractus solitarius.

Special visceral afferent component: *the nucleus of the tractus solitarius* (Fig 56)

Pseudo-unipolar nerve cells in the inferior glossopharyngeal ganglion receive, via their peripheral process, gustatory sensations from the post-sulcal tongue

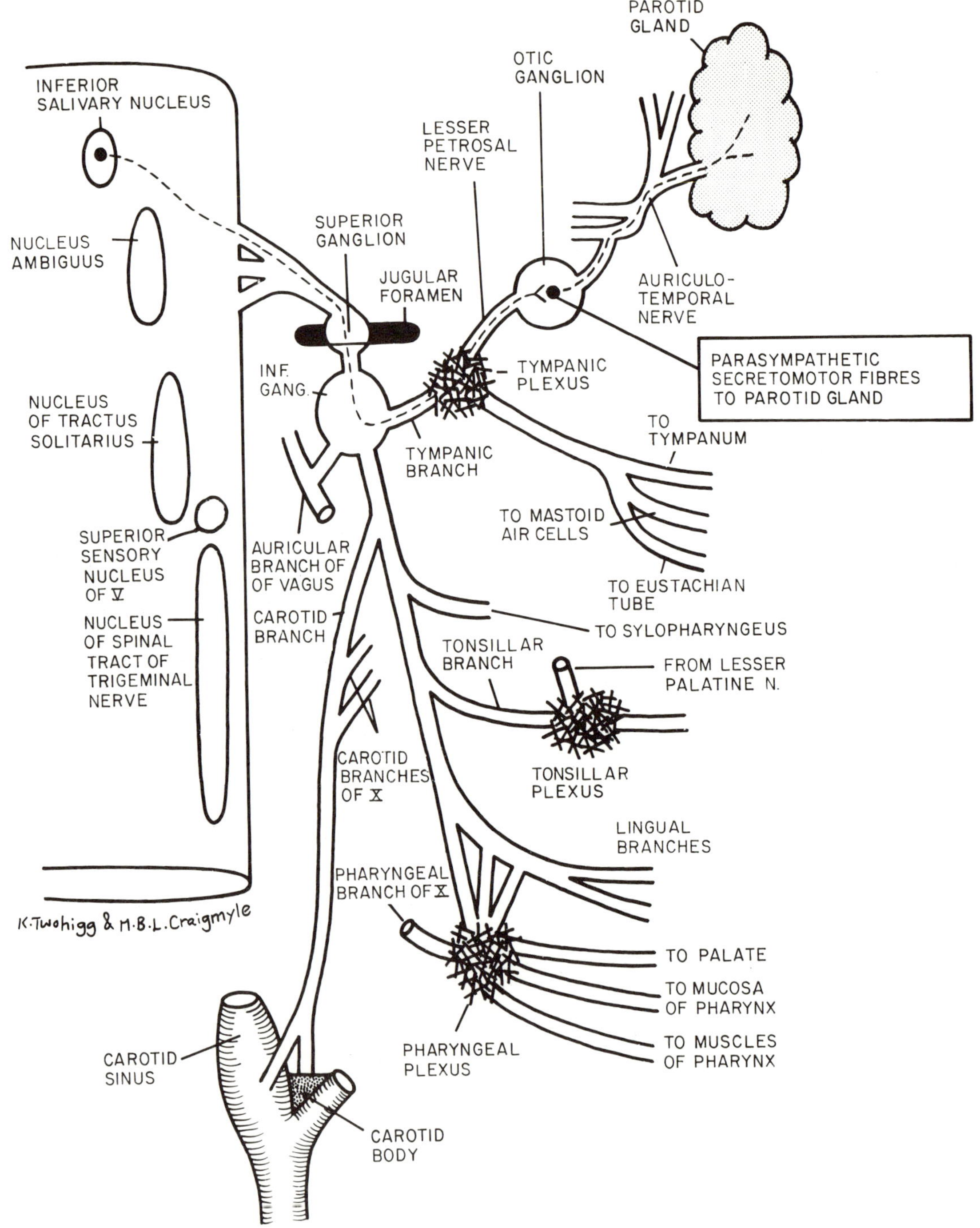

Fig 53   The distribution of the glossopharyngeal nerve: the general visceral efferent component.

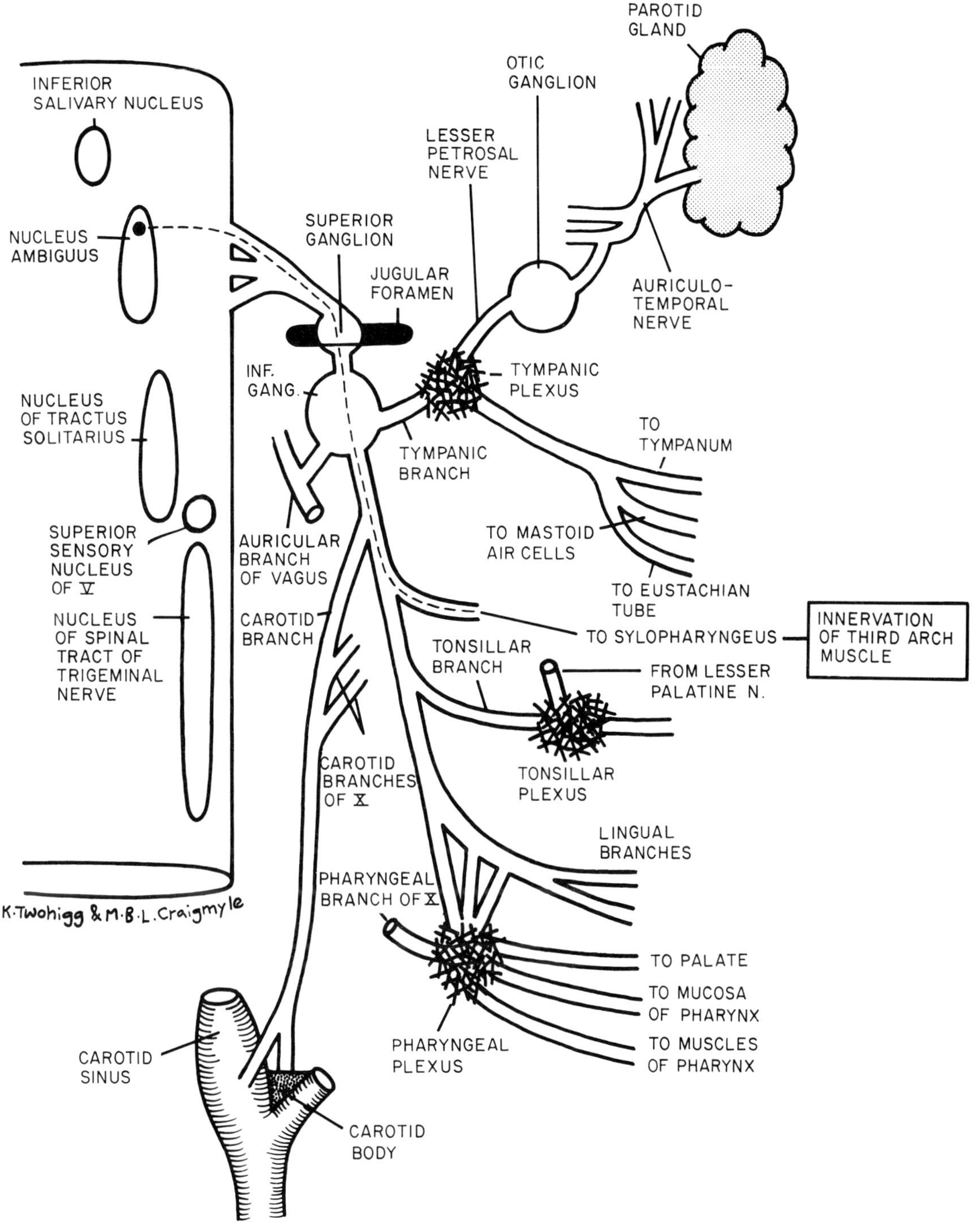

Fig 54 The distribution of the glossopharyngeal nerve: the special visceral efferent component.

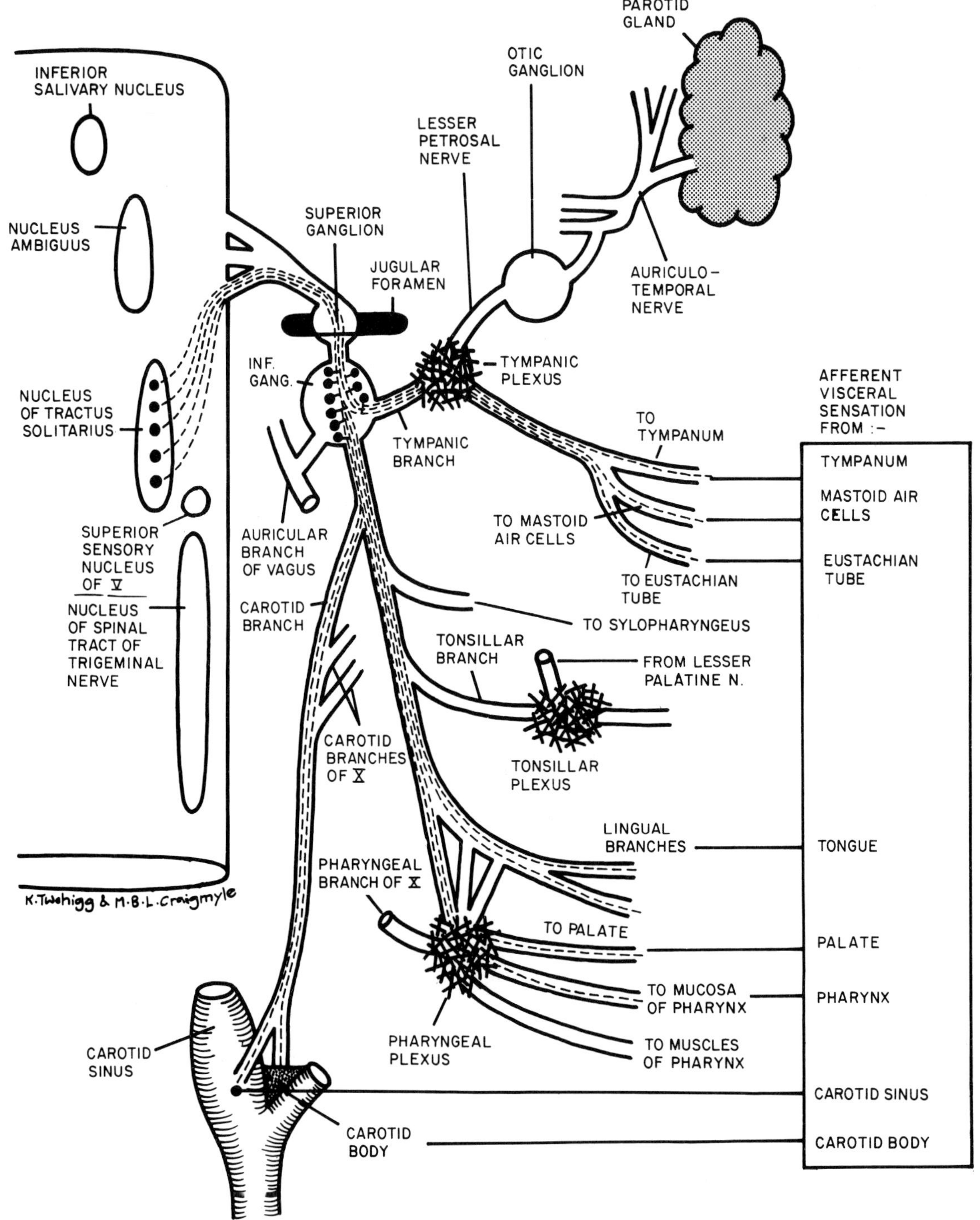

Fig 55   The distribution of the glossopharyngeal nerve: the general visceral afferent component.

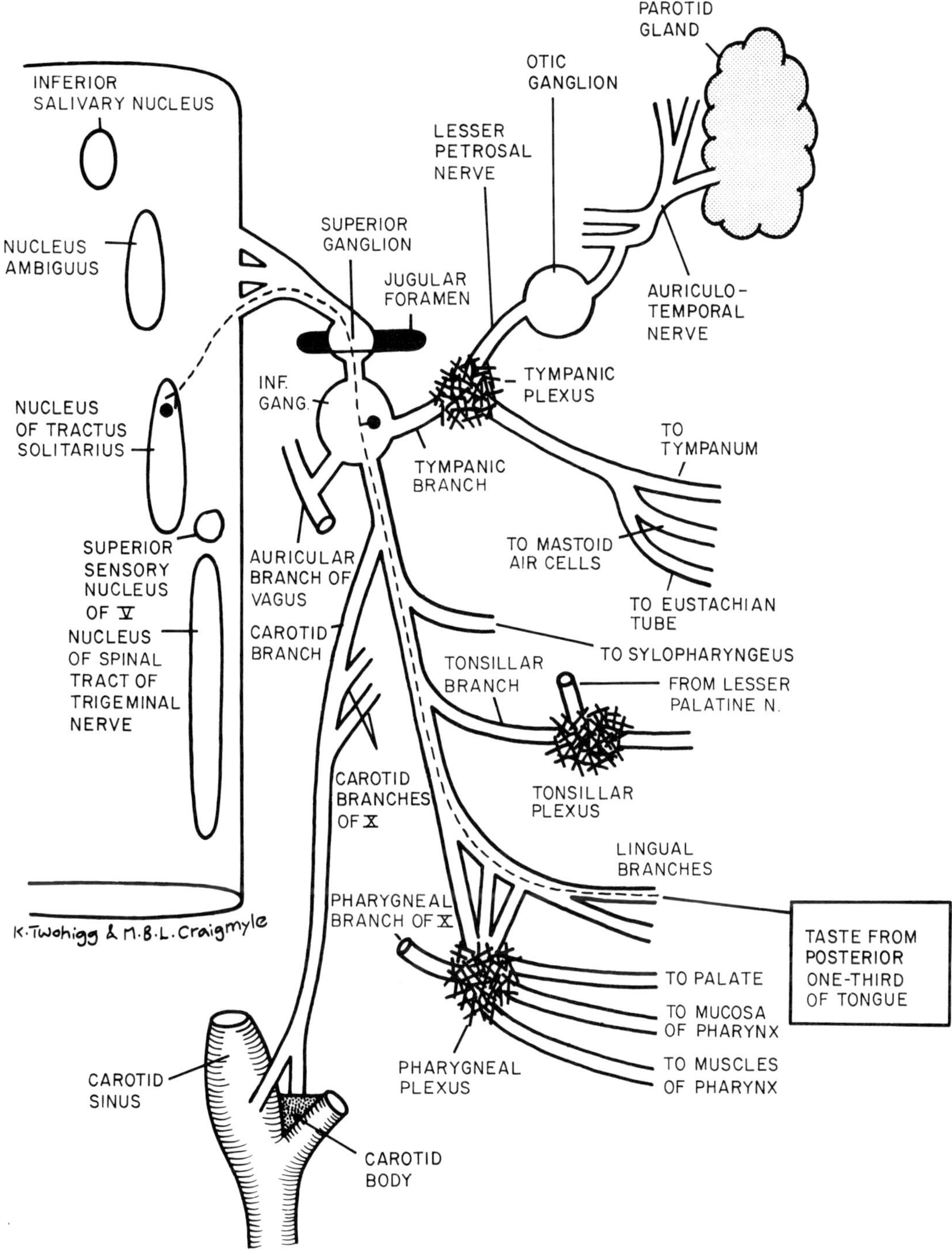

Fig 56 The distribution of the glossopharyngeal nerve: the special visceral afferent component.

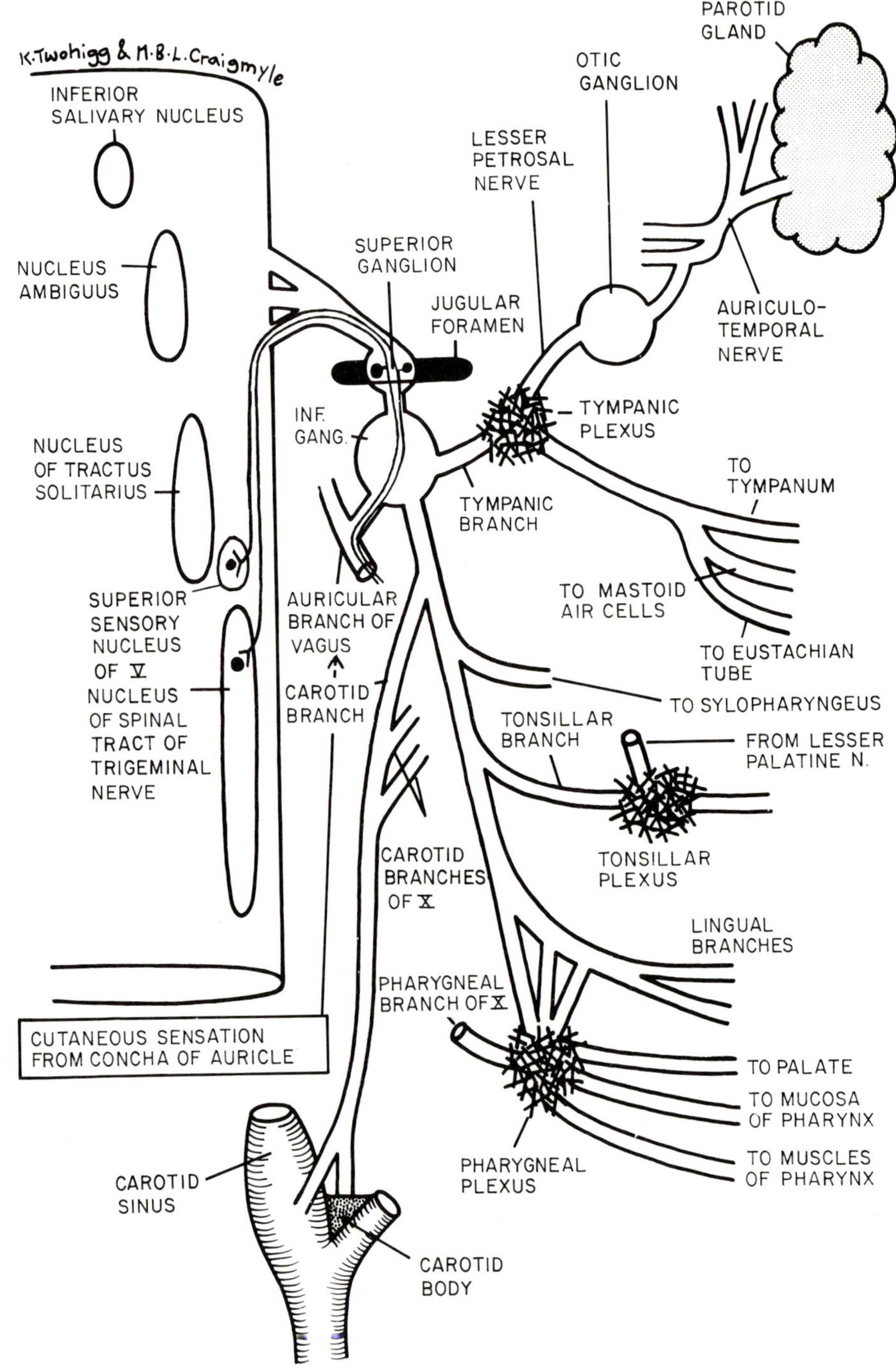

Fig 57 The distribution of the glossopharyngeal nerve: the general somatic afferent component.

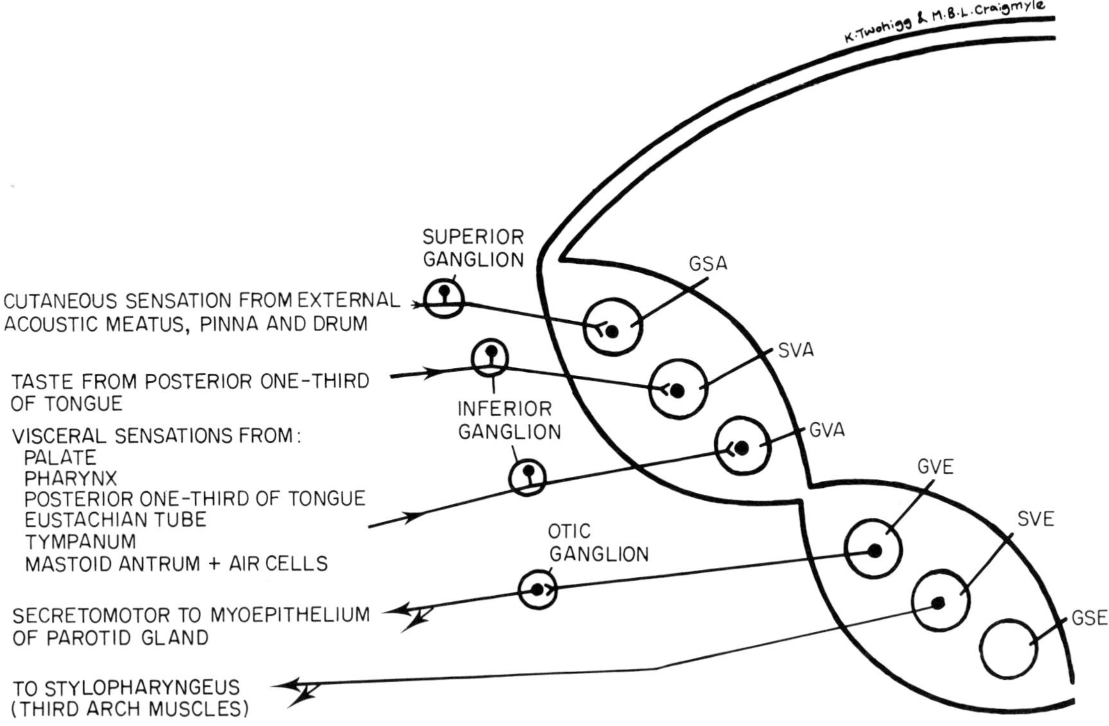

Fig 58 Summary of the nuclear connections of the glossopharyngeal nerve.

and the vallate papillae. Their central processes end in the upper part of the nucleus of the tractus solitarius.

General somatic afferent component: *the superior sensory nucleus and the spinal nucleus of the trigeminal nerve* (Fig 57)

The glossopharyngeal nerve sends, from its inferior ganglion, a communicating twig to the auricular branch of the vagus. The two nerves share, with the facial nerve, cutaneous sensations from the auricle and the external acoustic meatus. The pseudo-unipolar nerve cell bodies lie in the superior ganglion. Their central processes will terminate either in the superior sensory nucleus of the trigeminal nerve (in the case of tactile sensations) or in the nucleus of the spinal tract of the trigeminal nerve (in the case of thermal and painful sensations).

The nuclear connections of the glossopharyngeal nerve are summarised in Figure 58.

LESIONS OF THE GLOSSOPHARYNGEAL NERVE

These result in loss of general sensation from the posterior third of the tongue and from the pharynx, and in loss of taste in the posterior third of the tongue. Neuralgia of the nerve occurs in the ear and throat, and is precipitated or exacerbated by swallowing. The painful attacks are brief, as are those of trigeminal neuralgia, from which the syndrome has to be distinguished. Tumours of the pharyngeal wall or tonsil may be the cause. In any glossopharyngeal lesion, the motor loss is undetectable since only stylopharyngeus is affected.

SITES OF LESION

The commonest site of a glossopharyngeal nerve lesion is at or near the jugular foramen and the vagus and accessory nerves are then usually involved (Vernet's syndrome). The causes are listed in the chapter on the vagus nerve (Chapter 13).

13

THE VAGUS NERVE

ORIGIN, COURSE AND DISTRIBUTION (Fig 59)

The vagus nerve arises from the medulla oblongata, by eight to ten rootlets, from the interval between the olive and inferior cerebellar peduncle (Fig 19). It passes below the flocculus of the cerebellum to enter the jugular foramen in company with the glossopharyngeal and accessory nerves and the sigmoid and inferior petrosal sinuses. After traversing the foramen the vagus nerve exhibits two gangliform swellings, a small round superior ganglion (which contains the pseudo-unipolar cell bodies of general somatic afferent neurones) and a large oval inferior ganglion (which contains the pseudo-unipolar cells subserving general visceral afferent and special visceral afferent sensations). The superior ganglion of the vagus gives rise to meningeal and auricular branches. The inferior ganglion of the vagus gives rise to a pharyngeal branch, to minute and variable branches to the carotid body, and to the superior laryngeal nerve: the inferior ganglion is joined by the cranial accessory nerve. The vagus nerve enters the carotid sheath and runs behind, and between, the internal jugular vein and the *internal* carotid artery as far as the upper border of the thyroid cartilage: below this level and as far as the root of the neck, the vagus lies deep to, and between, the internal jugular vein and the *common* carotid artery. During its course in the neck it gives off upper and lower cervical cardiac branches. From this point on it is necessary to describe the two vagus nerves separately because their courses differ on the two sides.

The *right vagus nerve* passes in front of the first part of the subclavian artery, giving off the recurrent laryngeal nerve as it does so. It enters the superior mediastinum of the thorax, passing behind the right brachiocephalic vein before coming to lie to the right of the trachea, between it and the pleura and lung. The nerve then runs posteromedial to the right brachiocephalic vein and the superior vena cava. It gives branches to the oesophagus and trachea, to the anterior pulmonary plexus and thoracic cardiac branches. The nerve then passes behind the hilum of the right lung and breaks up into a plexus which, with twigs from the second, third and fourth ganglia of the thoracic sympathetic chain, forms the right posterior pulmonary plexus. Caudally, the plexus gives rise to two or three branches which, with a branch from the left vagus, descend dorsal to the oesophagus as the posterior oesophageal plexus. The plexus forms a trunk which contains fibres of both vagus nerves and which enters the abdomen through the oesophageal

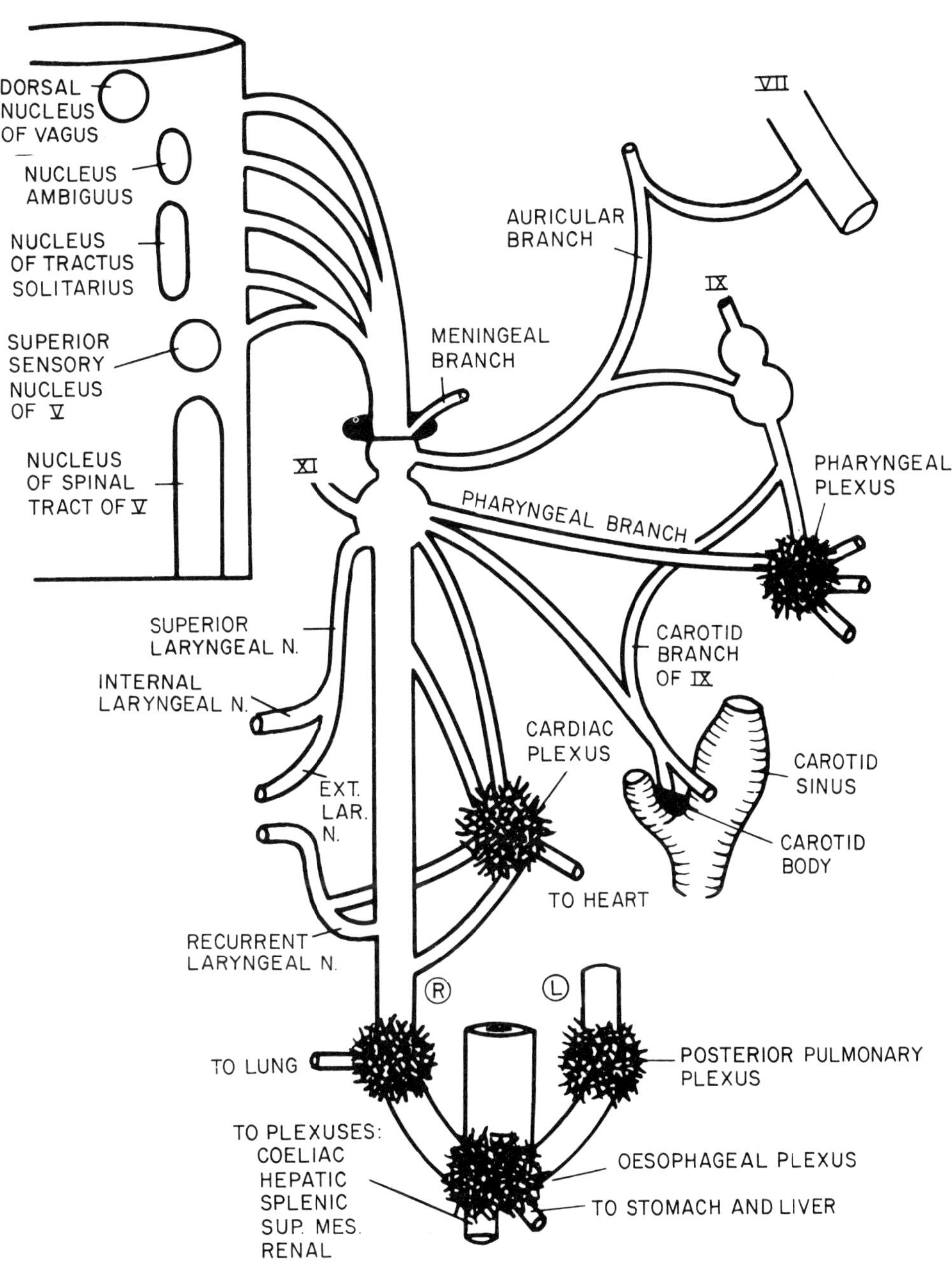

Fig 59 The distribution of the vagus nerve.

opening in the diaphragm before dividing into large coeliac and small gastric branches. The coeliac branch sends twigs to the hepatic, splenic, renal, suprarenal and superior mesenteric plexuses but its main contribution is to the coeliac plexus. The gastric branch supplies the postero-superior aspect of the body of the stomach. The abdominal portions of the vagus nerves in Figure 59 are shown in very simplified form.

The left vagus

This nerve enters the thorax between the left subclavian and left common carotid arteries, and behind the left brachio-cephalic vein. In the superior mediastinum it passes to the left of the arch of the aorta, giving off here the left recurrent laryngeal nerve and being crossed in turn by the left phrenic nerve and the left superior inter-costal vein. It passes behind the root of the left lung and breaks up into the posterior pulmonary plexus (which is joined by branches from the second to fourth left thoracic sympathetic ganglia inclusive). Two branches descend, from this plexus, on the front of the oesophagus where they are joined by a branch from the right vagus to form the anterior oesophageal plexus. This plexus then forms a single trunk which contains fibres of both vagi and which enters the abdomen through the oesophageal opening in the diaphragm anterior to the oesophagus. In the abdomen the nerve supplies the cardia of the stomach before dividing into right and left branches. The right branch sends components to:

the liver via the lesser omentum and porta hepatis;
to the pylorus and head of the pancreas and the first and second parts of the duodenum;
to the anterosuperior part of the body of the stomach; and
to the lesser curvature of the stomach.

The left branch is distributed to the anterosuperior surface of the stomach.

The abdominal portions of the vagus nerves are simplified in Figure 59.

SUMMARY OF THE BRANCHES OF THE VAGUS

1   In the jugular foramen: from the superior ganglion

   (a)   meningeal branch
   (b)   auricular branch

2   In the neck: from the inferior ganglion

   (a)   pharyngeal branch
   (b)   superior laryngeal nerve
   (c)   carotid body branches
   (d)   recurrent laryngeal nerve (right vagus only)

3   In the thorax

   (i)   recurrent laryngeal nerve (left vagus only)
   (ii)   cardiac
   (iii)   pulmonary
   (iv)   oesophageal

4   In the abdomen

   (i)   gastric
   (ii)   hepatic
   (iii)   coeliac
   (iv)   renal

The *meningeal branch* arises from the superior ganglion. It is distributed to the dura of the posterior cranial fossa. It is probably vasomotor sympathetic (from the superior cervical sympathetic ganglion) and sensory from the upper cervical nerves (which communicate with the vagus).

The *auricular branch* arises from the superior ganglion of the vagus, and receives twigs from (1) the inferior ganglion of the glossopharyngeal nerve and (2) from the facial nerve. The nerve enters the small mastoid canaliculus in the lateral wall of the jugular fossa. This canal cuts across the canal in the petrous temporal for the facial nerve, and the vagal and facial nerves here communicate. The auricular branch of the vagus emerges on the base of the skull through the tympano-mastoid fissure. It is distributed to:

the skin on the cranial surface of the pinna,
the postero-inferior wall of the external acoustic meatus, and
the adjoining part of the outer surface of the tympanic membrane.

The *pharyngeal branch* of the vagus arises from the inferior vagal ganglion. It passes between the internal and external carotid arteries to reach the upper edge of the middle constrictor muscle of the pharynx where it forms the pharyngeal plexus with the pharyngeal branches of the glossopharyngeal nerve, and filaments from the cervical sympathetic trunk.

The *branch to the carotid body* is very variable in its origin, since it may arise from the inferior ganglion or the pharyngeal branch of the vagus. The nerve may have several branches. It communicates with the carotid branch of the glossopharyngeal nerve which is distributed to the carotid body and the carotid sinus.

The *superior laryngeal nerve* arises from the inferior vagal ganglion. It descends on the side wall of the pharynx medial to the internal carotid artery. It divides into a large internal and a tiny external laryngeal branch. The *internal laryngeal nerve* enters the laryngeal wall by piercing the thyrohyoid membrane. It is sensory to the mucosa of the larynx above the vocal folds, and to the mucosa of the pyriform fossa, vallecula and the epiglottis. The *external laryngeal nerve* runs down on the inferior constrictor after passing under the sternothyroid. It supplies the cricothyroid muscle, and the inferior constrictor of the pharynx.

The *recurrent laryngeal nerve* arises differently on the two sides. On the *right* it arises from the vagus in front of the first part of the right subclavian artery, and turns below and behind that artery to gain the side of the trachea. On the *left* the recurrent laryngeal nerve is given off as the vagus crosses the aortic arch and turns below and behind the vessel and behind the ligamentum arteriosum to gain the side of the trachea.

The recurrent laryngeal nerves on each side give off cardiac branches to the deep cardiac plexus and ascend in the groove between the oesophagus and the trachea, passing behind the lobe of the thyroid gland to enter the larynx below the lower border of the inferior constrictor muscle of the pharynx. They give branches to all the muscles of the larynx except cricothyroid, and are sensory to the mucosa of the larynx below the level of the vocal folds. The nerves also supply mucosa and muscle of both trachea and oesophagus, and the inferior constrictor muscle.

The thoracic cardiac branches

These are given off as two or three twigs which join the deep cardiac plexus.

The *pulmonary branches* are grouped in anterior and posterior sets and form, with sympathetic filaments from the second to fifth thoracic ganglia inclusive, the anterior and posterior pulmonary plexuses. From these the mucosa and musculature of the broncho-pulmonary tree are supplied.

The oesophageal branches

These are given off above and especially below the lung hilum. They form the oesophageal plexus from which the mucosa and musculature of the oesophagus derives its supply.

The gastric branches

The postero-inferior aspect of the stomach is supplied mainly by the right and the anterosuperior aspect mainly by the left vagus.

The *hepatic branches* arise from both vagi.

The *renal branches* arise from both vagi and form the renal plexus. They are mainly vasomotor to the renal vessels.

The *coeliac branches* join the coeliac plexus. From this plexus the portions of alimentary canal of foregut and midgut origin are supplied, ie. small gut, ascending colon and first two-thirds of the transverse colon, spleen, pancreas, liver and gall bladder. In addition the coeliac plexus supplies the kidneys, upper ureters and gonads.

THE DEEP CENTRAL CONNECTIONS OF THE VAGUS NERVE See Chapter 6

NUCLEAR CONNECTIONS OF THE VAGUS NERVE

General visceral efferent component: *the dorsal motor nucleus of the vagus* (Fig 60)

This nucleus supplies the smooth muscle of:

(i) The tracheobronchial tree,
(ii) The oesophagus, liver, spleen, stomach, gall bladder, ureter, small gut and the large gut as far as the junction of middle and distal thirds of the transverse colon.

The dorsal motor nucleus also supplies the cardiac muscle.

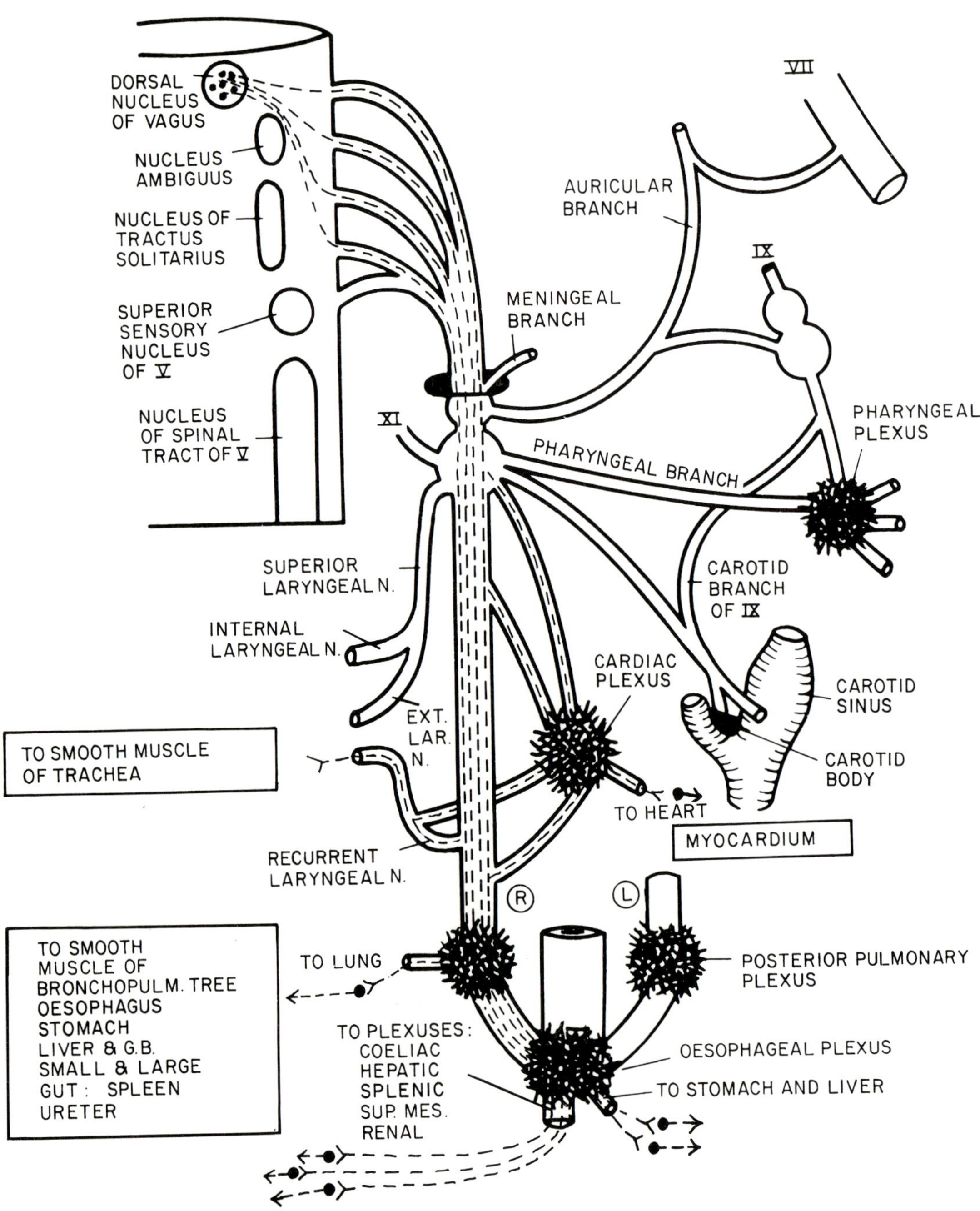

Fig 60   The distribution of the vagus nerve: the general visceral efferent component.

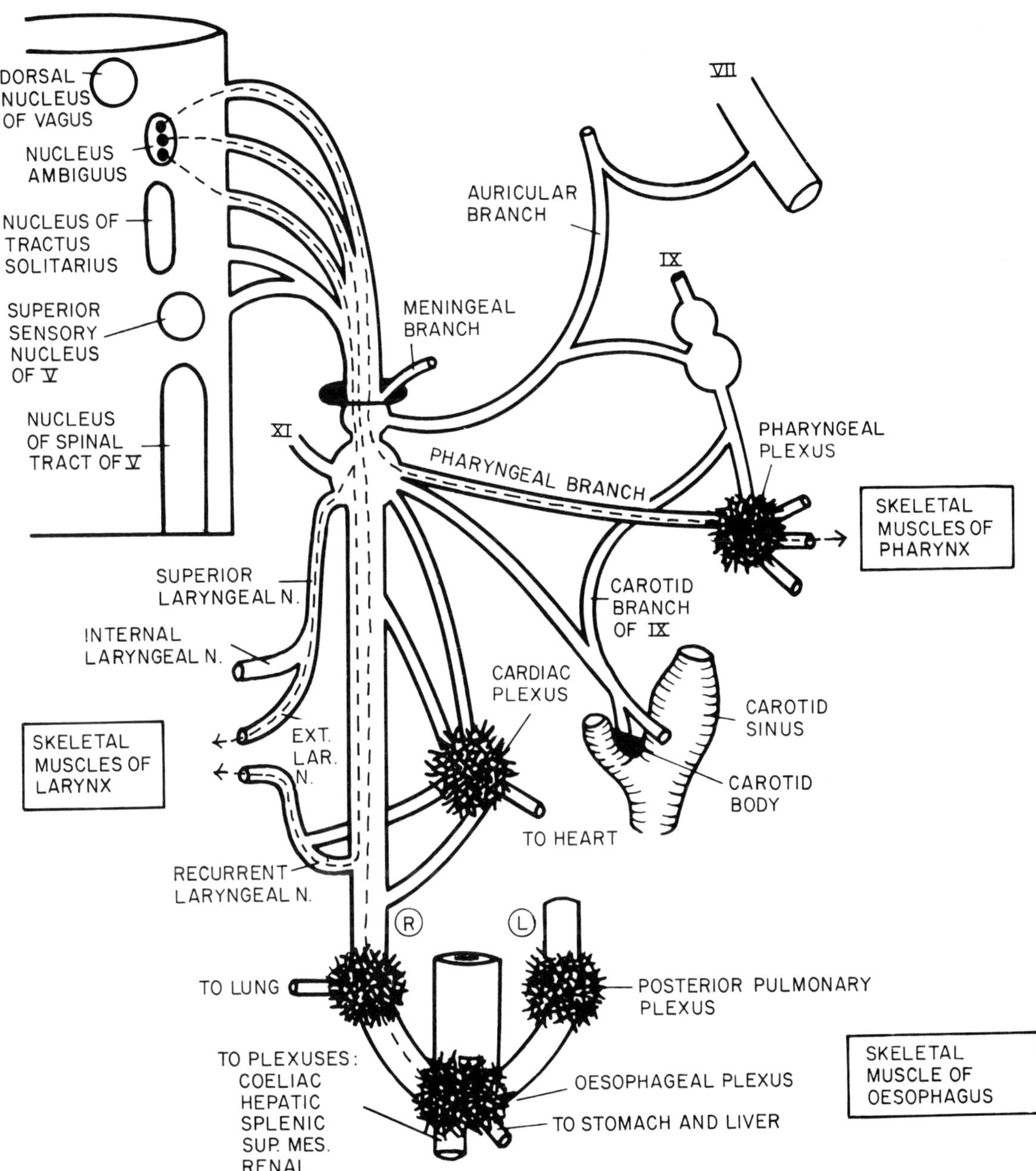

Fig 61 The distribution of the vagus nerve: the special visceral (branchial) efferent component.

Special visceral efferent component: *the nucleus ambiguus* (Fig 61)

The lower motor neurones in this (branchial efferent) nucleus furnish fibres to the glossopharyngeal nerve (for the supply of stylopharyngeus) and to the cranial accessory and vagus nerves. Since these two blend it is not possible to separate the skeletal muscles supplied by each. The two nerves collectively supply, via the pharyngeal plexus, the skeletal muscle of:

pharynx (except stylopharyngeus)
larynx
upper two-thirds of the oesophagus
palate (except tensor palati)

General visceral afferent component: *the nucleus of the tractus solitarius* (Fig 62)

The cell bodies in the *inferior* vagal ganglion are pseudo-unipolar. Their central processes terminate on the cells in the *lower* end of the nucleus of the tractus solitarius. Their distal processes bring visceral afferent sensations from:

tonsils	pancreas
palate	liver
larynx	gall bladder
oesophagus	kidneys
stomach	gonads
small gut	heart
most of large gut	carotid sinus
tracheobronchial tree	carotid body
spleen	

Special visceral afferent component: *the nucleus of the tractus solitarius* (Fig 63)

Taste sensations from the epiglottis are conveyed by the distal processes of the pseudo-unipolar nerve cells in the *inferior* vagal ganglion and reach the *upper* end of the nucleus of the tractus solitarius via their central processes.

General somatic afferent component: *the nucleus of the spinal tract and superior sensory nucleus of the trigeminal nerve* (Fig 64)

The ganglion cells in the *superior* vagal ganglion are pseudo-unipolar. Their peripheral processes receive cutaneous sensations from the pinna, the external acoustic meatus and the eardrum. Their central processes terminate in the nucleus of the spinal tract of, and in the superior sensory nucleus of, the trigeminal nerve.

The nuclear connections of the vagus nerve are summarised in Figure 65.

LESIONS OF THE VAGUS NERVE

The vagus nerve trunk is not damaged very commonly. The patient will complain of palpitation, constant vomiting and a feeling of suffocation. He will have tachycardia and a reduced respiratory rate. He will have paralysis of the soft palate, pharynx and larynx on the affected side. When asked to say 'Ah' the soft palate moves to the affected side.

Lesions of the vagus nerve in the lower part of the neck may affect the superior and recurrent laryngeal nerves, or only the latter. When both nerves are involved, there is complete anaesthesia of the larynx and complete inability to move the vocal folds on the affected side, so the voice is weak. When only the recurrent laryngeal nerve is involved, there is anaesthesia of the lower larynx and the voice is again weak. The superior laryngeal nerve alone may be damaged, with the result that loss of cricothyroid makes the voice hoarse and deep: the concomitant anaesthesia of the upper larynx allows of easy entry by foreign bodies, with resultant spasm of the glottis.

Vagal reflexes are common, some examples of which are:

coughing and perhaps even vomiting when the ear is swabbed or syringed;
eczema of the skin behind the ear causing sneezing;
brassy cough from pressure on the recurrent laryngeal nerve from such conditions as aneurysm of the aorta or enlargement of bronchial lymph nodes.

SITES OF LESION

I.   *In the brain stem*

(a)   Posterior inferior cerebellar artery thrombosis
(b)   Encephalitis
(c)   Medullary tumours

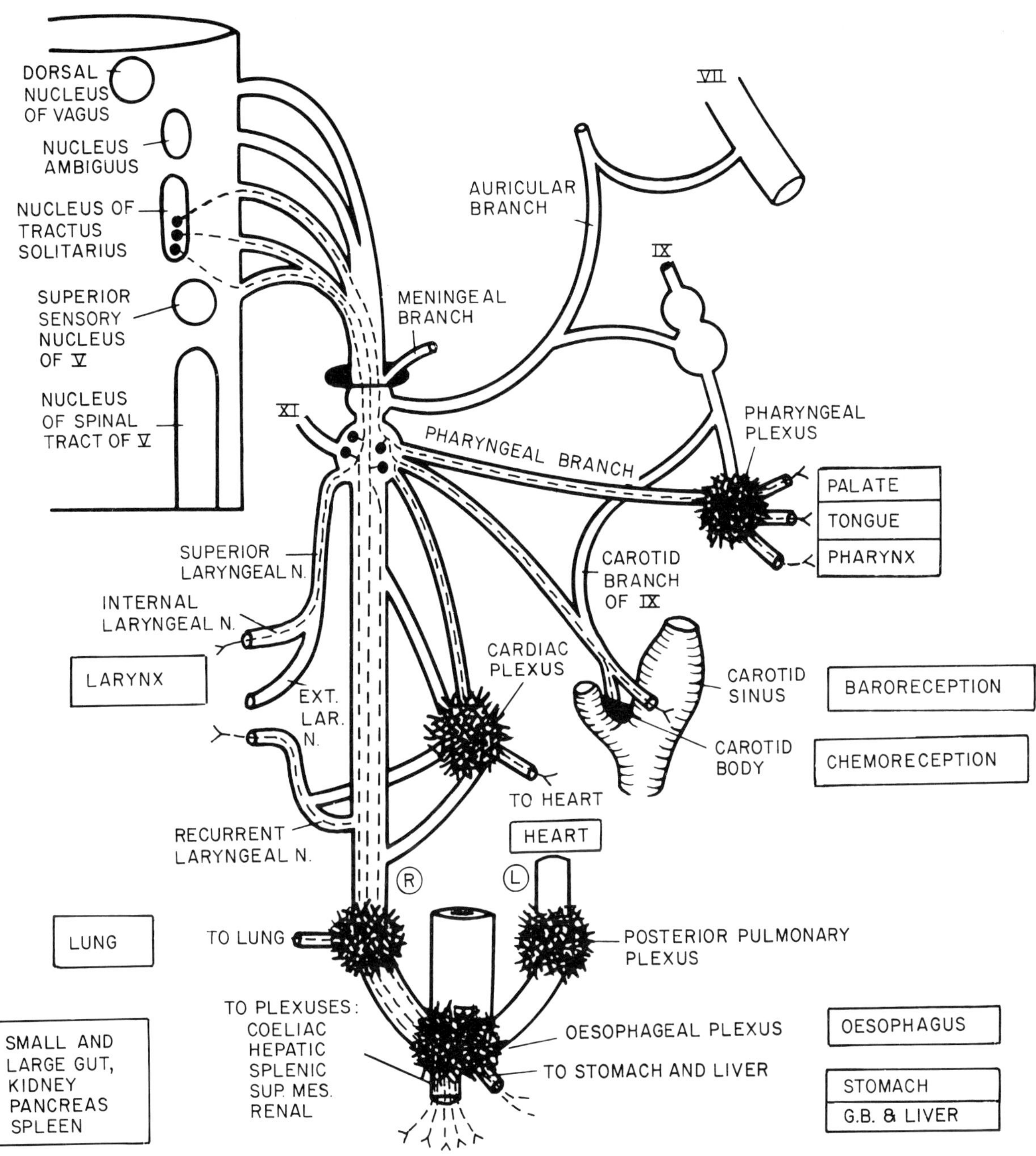

Fig 62 The distribution of the vagus nerve: the general visceral afferent component.

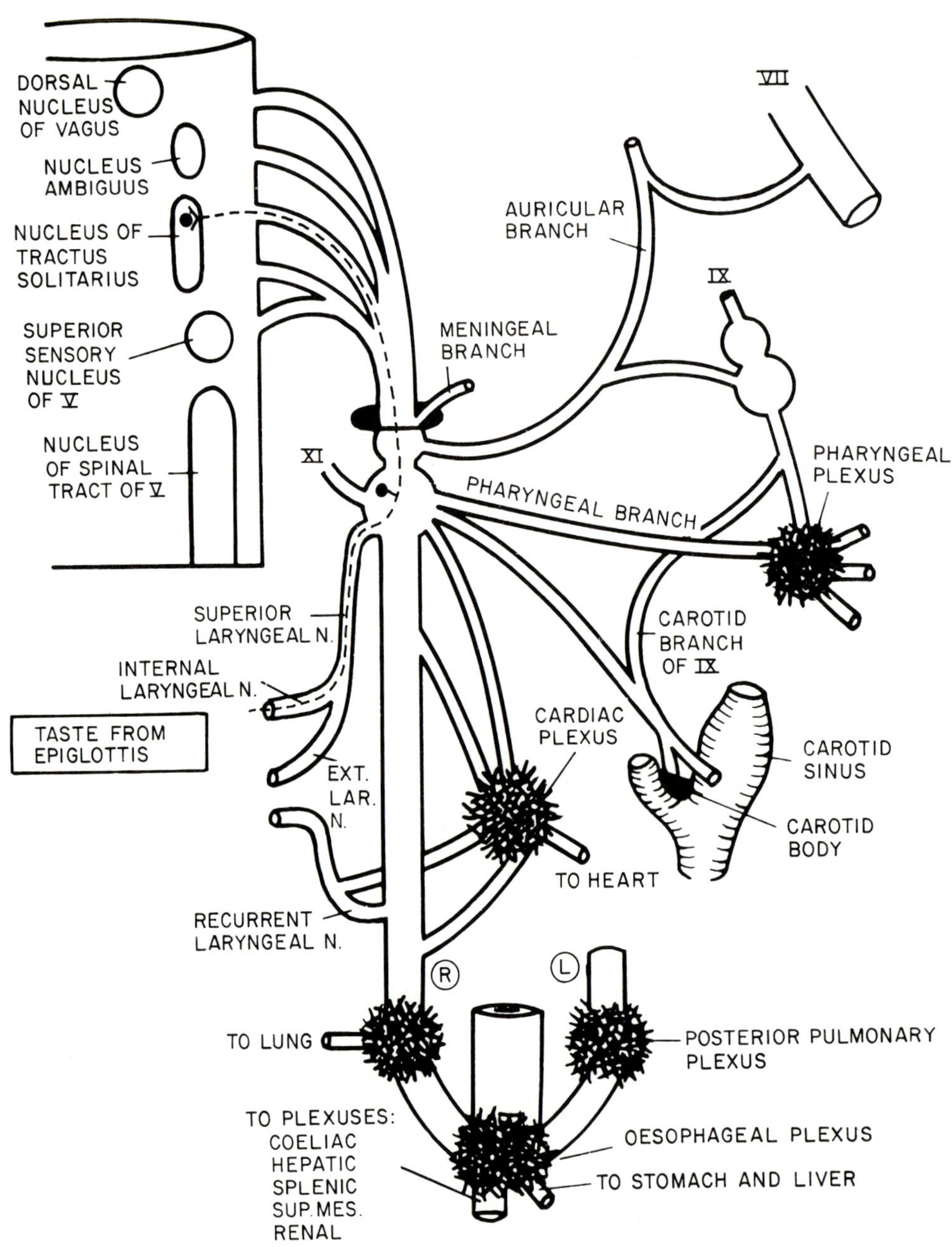

Fig 63   The distribution of the vagus nerve: the special visceral afferent (taste) component.

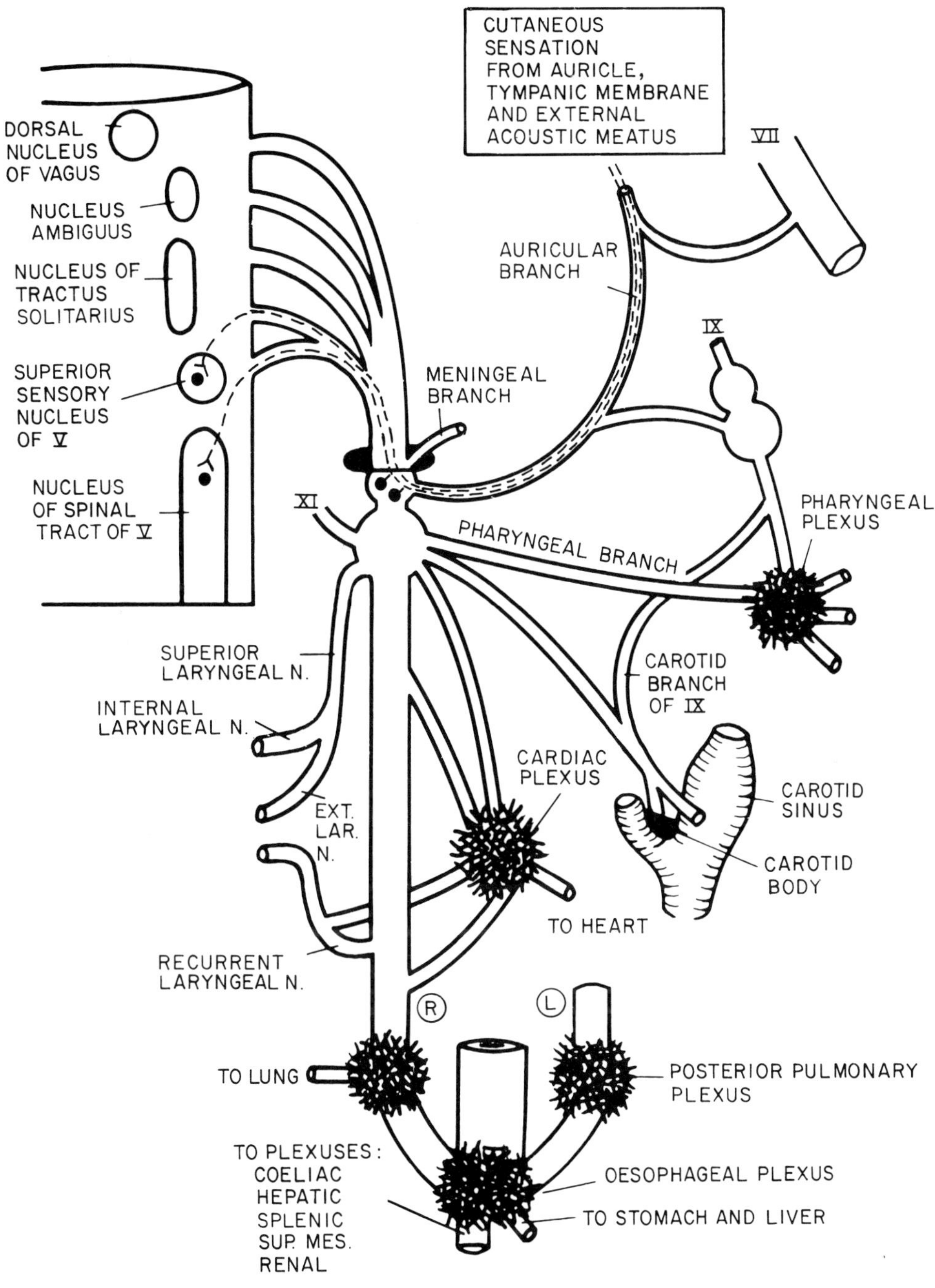

Fig 64   The distribution of the vagus nerve: the general somatic afferent component.

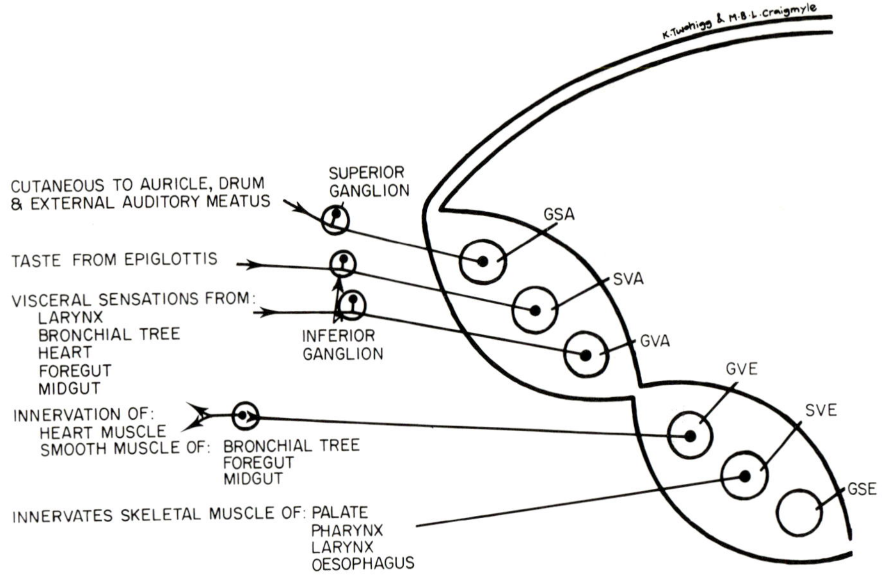

Fig 65   Summary of the nuclear connections of the vagus nerve.

(d)   Syringobulbia
(e)   Tabes dorsalis
(f)   Poliomyelitis
(g)   Motor neurone disease

II.   *In the cerebellopontine angle*

(a)   Cerebellar tumours
(b)   Syphilis
(c)   Middle ear infections
(d)   Pontine glioma
(e)   Aneurysm of the basilar artery
(f)   Neuroma of nerves VII, VIII, IX, XI or XII
(g)   Carcinoma of the nasopharynx
(h)   Meningiomata
(i)   Epidermoid tumours
(j)   Neurofibromata
(k)   Ectopic glomus tumours

The following observations are important:

1   If the vagus lesion is being produced by a tumour of one of the other cranial nerves in the cerebellopontine angle (i.e. of VII, VIII, IX, XI or XII) then a lesion of that nerve will be superimposed on the clinical picture.

In fact, if V or VII are involved the lesion must be *inside* the skull because no lesion outside the skull could produce a combination of this type.

2   The cervical sympathetic ascends to the jugular foramen: if there is a Horner's syndrome present, the lesion must be outside the skull.

Several syndromes are recognised:

Vernet's syndrome	— IX, X and XI involved
Schmidt's syndrome	— X and XI involved
Hughlings-Jackson syndrome	— X, XI and XII involved
Collet-Secard syndrome	— IX, X, XI and XII involved
Villaret's syndrome	— IX, X, XI and XII involved, with Horner's syndrome superimposed, ie. a lesion below the jugular foramen affecting the cervical sympathetic in addition.

14

THE ACCESSORY NERVE

ORIGIN, COURSE AND DISTRIBUTION (Fig 66)

This nerve arises by a small cranial root referred to often as the cranial accessory nerve, and a large spinal root (spinal accessory nerve). The *cranial root* arises from the medulla oblongata below the vagus as four or five fine rootlets (Fig 19). It joins the spinal root near the jugular foramen to form the accessory nerve. The *spinal root* arises as a series of some 12 rootlets from the side of the upper portion of the cervical spinal cord: the rootlets emerge midway between the dorsal and ventral roots of the upper five cervical nerves. The rootlets unite to form a single trunk which ascends in the subarachnoid space behind the ligamentum denticulatum (Fig 19). It enters the skull through the foramen magnum, and bends laterally to join the cranial root. The accessory nerve enters the jugular foramen and at its exit from the foramen separates into its cranial and spinal components. The cranial component crosses over the inferior ganglion of the vagus, at which point it joins that nerve. It is distributed through the pharyngeal and recurrent laryngeal branches of the vagus for the most part. The spinal root runs laterally behind (occasionally in front of) the internal jugular vein, crossing the transverse process of the atlas in so doing. The spinal accessory nerve

then descends obliquely in the neck surrounded by the retropharyngeal lymph nodes and passes deep to the styloid process, and the posterior belly of the digastric and stylohyoid muscles. It reaches the deep surface of the sternocleidomastoid muscle, accompanied by the superior sternocleidomastoid branch of the occipital artery. It enters the muscle, supplying it (along with branches from the second cervical nerve). The accessory nerve emerges from the posterior border of the muscle, near its middle, and crosses the posterior triangle of the neck in its fascial roof. It passes under the anterior border of trapezius about two inches above the clavicle and forms the subtrapezoid plexus with branches from the anterior primary rami of the third and fourth cervical nerves. The trapezius muscle is innervated by this plexus.

DEEP CENTRAL CONNECTIONS OF THE ACCESSORY NERVE See Chapter 6

NUCLEAR CONNECTIONS OF SPINAL ROOT

General somatic efferent or special visceral efferent component (Fig 67)

The spinal root originates from the spinal nucleus, which

85

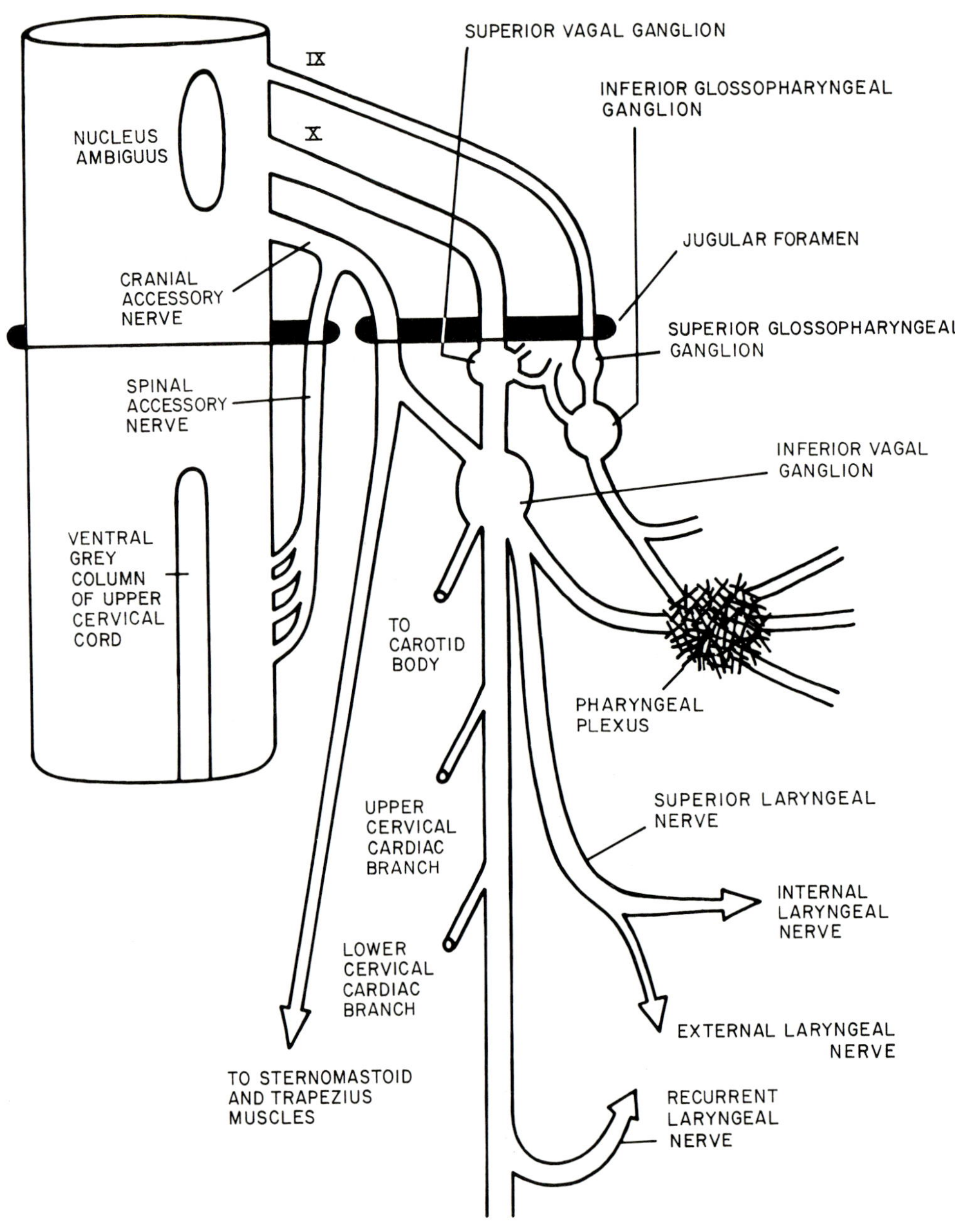

Fig 66   The distribution of the accessory nerve.

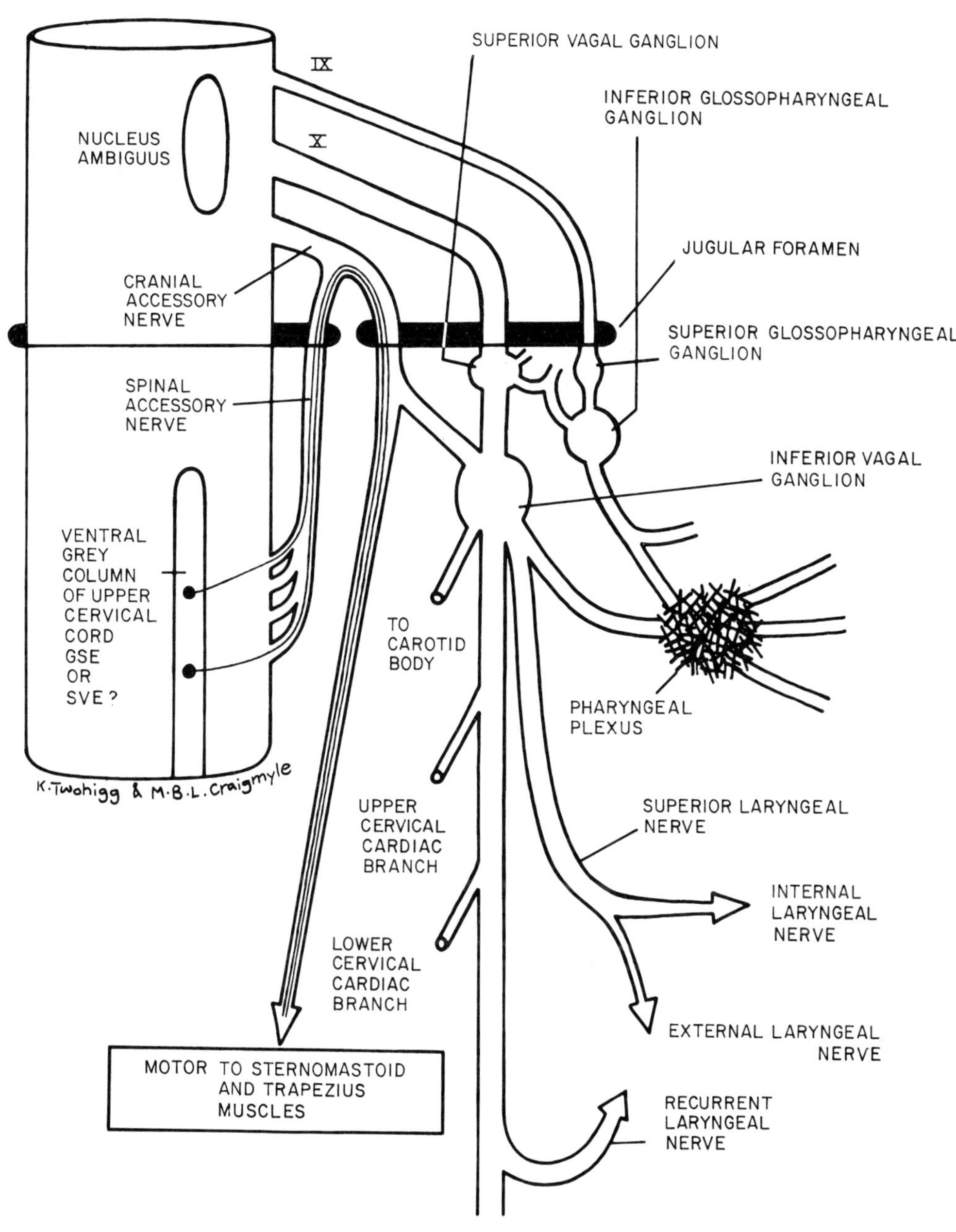

Fig 67   The distribution of the accessory nerve: the spinal component (GSE or SVE).

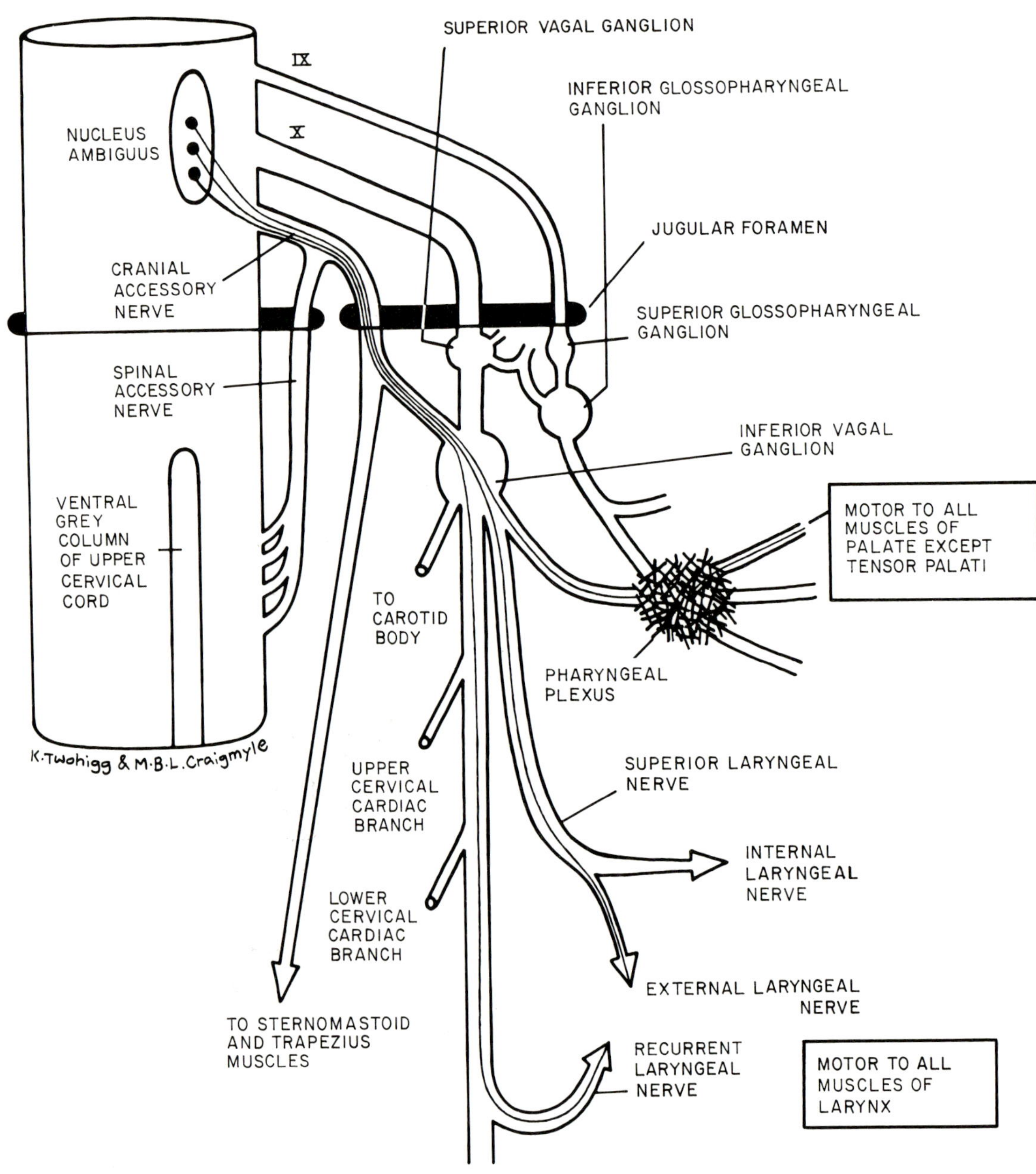

Fig 68 The distribution of the accessory nerve: the cranial component — special visceral efferent.

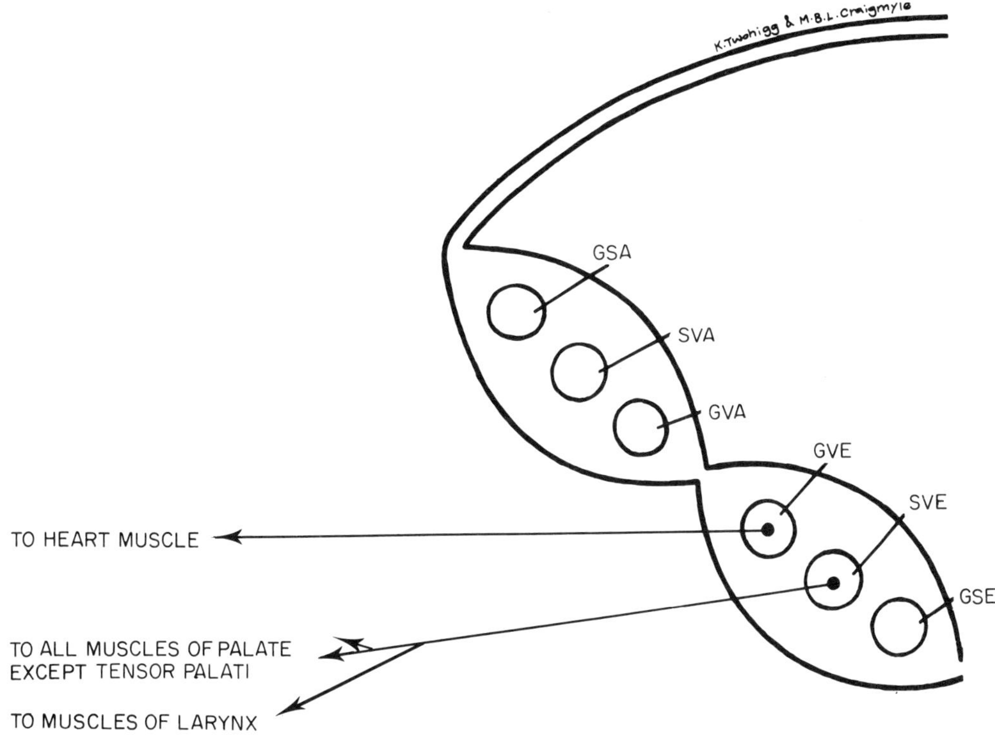

Fig 69   Summary of the nuclear connections of the cranial accessory nerve.

lies in the lateral part of the anterior grey column of the spinal cord. The nature of this nucleus will be GSE or SVE depending on the developmental origin of the sternocleidomastoid and trapezius muscles (to which it is motor). If these muscles are derived from the occipital somites then the spinal nucleus is general somatic efferent: if these muscles originate from pharyngeal arch mesoderm, then the nucleus is special visceral efferent. The controversy may never be resolved.

NUCLEAR CONNECTIONS OF THE CRANIAL ROOT

Special visceral (branchial) efferent component: *the nucleus ambiguus* (Fig 68)

The axons from the lower motor neurones of the lower end of the nucleus ambiguus leave the cranial accessory nerve and join the vagus to be distributed:

1   via the pharyngeal branch of the vagus and the pharyngeal plexus to the skeletal muscles of the palate (except tensor palati) and,
2   via the superior and recurrent laryngeal nerves to the skeletal muscles of the larynx.

General visceral efferent component: *the dorsal nucleus of the vagus*

Some fibres from this nucleus are believed to join the cranial accessory nerve and be distributed to the myocardium via the cardiac branches of the vagus.

The nuclear connections of the accessory nerve are presented in summary in Figure 69.

LESIONS OF THE SPINAL ACCESSORY NERVE

Damage to the spinal accessory nerve results in paralysis of sternocleidomastoid and trapezius: the patient cannot shrug his shoulder on the affected side nor turn his head to the unaffected side. The nerve may be irritated by inflamed lymph nodes (retropharyngeal or deep cervical) with resultant wry neck (torticollis). If the spinal accessory nerve is irritated within the central nervous system, chronic spasm of sternocleidomastoid and trapezius (spasmodic torticollis) ensues.

In operative procedures for excision of the deep cervical nodes in the posterior triangle of the neck, the nerve must be secured at the outset.

SITES OF LESION OF THE CRANIAL ACCESSORY NERVE

See under vagus nerve, Chapter 13.

15

THE HYPOGLOSSAL NERVE

ORIGIN, COURSE AND DISTRIBUTION (Fig 70)

The hypoglossal nerve arises as a series of about half-a-dozen rootlets from the anterior aspect of the medulla oblongata between the olive and the pyramid. The rootlets pass behind the vertebral artery and form two roots which pass through the anterior condylar (hypoglossal) canal and unite just outside the base of the skull to form the hypoglossal nerve. Here it gives off a *meningeal branch.* The nerve initially is deep to, and then passes behind, the glossopharyngeal and vagus nerves to gain the interval between the internal jugular vein and the internal carotid artery. It half-spirals round the inferior vagal ganglion and then descends vertically in the back of the carotid sheath between the two great vessels and superficial to the vagus nerve. It is here joined by a twig from the first cervical nerve. After passing deep to the stylohyoid and the posterior belly of the digastric muscle, it bends sharply forwards, hooking round the inferior sternocleidomastoid branch of the occipital artery. Here it gives off its *descending branch.* The hypoglossal nerve then crosses in succession the internal and external carotid and lingual arteries, being crossed by the facial vein. It here gives off the *nerve to the thyrohyoid.* It now runs forwards and upwards on

the hyoglossus muscle, which it supplies, before passing deep to the digastric tendon, the stylohyoid and the mylohyoid: superior to it at this stage are the deep part of the submandibular gland, its duct, and the lingual nerve. The nerve then passes on to the surface of genioglossus, the substance of which it enters. It supplies this muscle and runs in its substance to the tip of the tongue. It supplies all the intrinsic muscles of the tongue, and hyoglossus, styloglossus and genioglossus of the extrinsic group of tongue muscles.

The *meningeal branch* reaches the posterior cranial fossa via the anterior condylar canal. It supplies the diploe of the occipital bone, the dura of occipital and inferior petrosal sinuses and the dura of the posterior cranial fossa. The fibres in this branch are derived in all probability from the upper cervical nerves and the superior cervical sympathetic ganglion, all of which communicate with the hypoglossal nerve.

The *descending branch* (N. descendens hypoglossi) runs, in succession, in the adventitial sheaths in front of the internal and common carotid arteries. It gives a branch to the superior belly of the omohyoid muscle before forming a loop — ansa cervicalis — with the descending cervical nerve (N. descendens cervicalis) which is derived from the second and third cervical

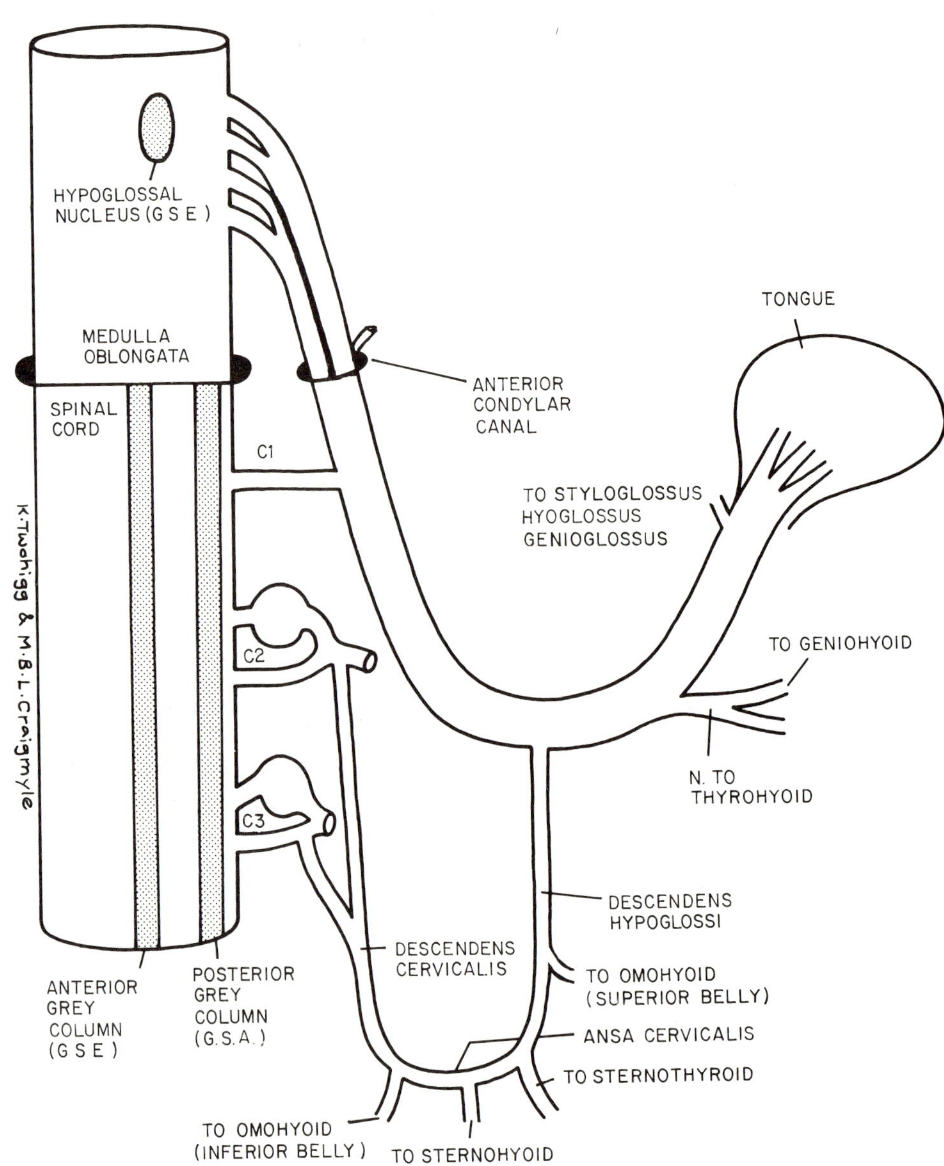

Fig 70   The distribution of the hypoglossal nerve.

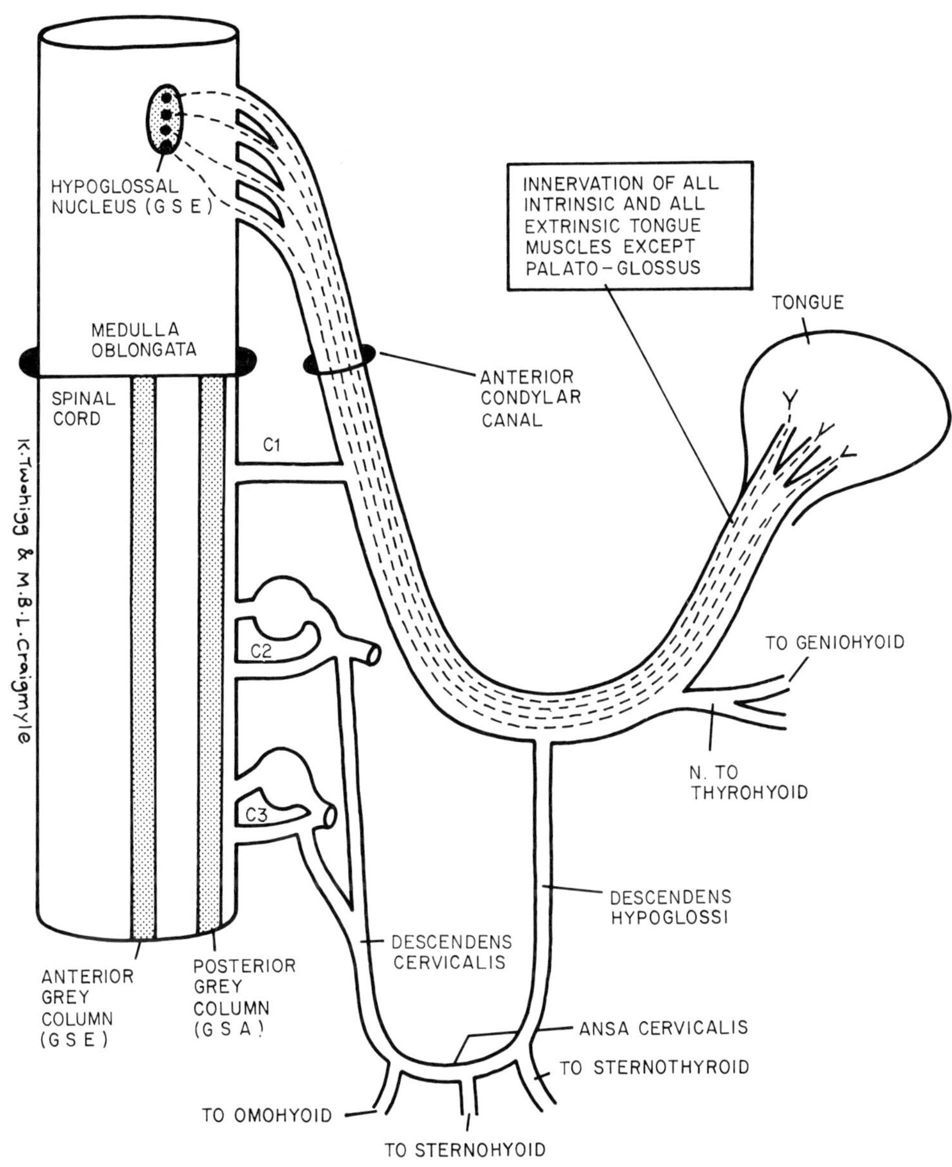

Fig 71 The distribution of the hypoglossal nerve: the general somatic efferent component.

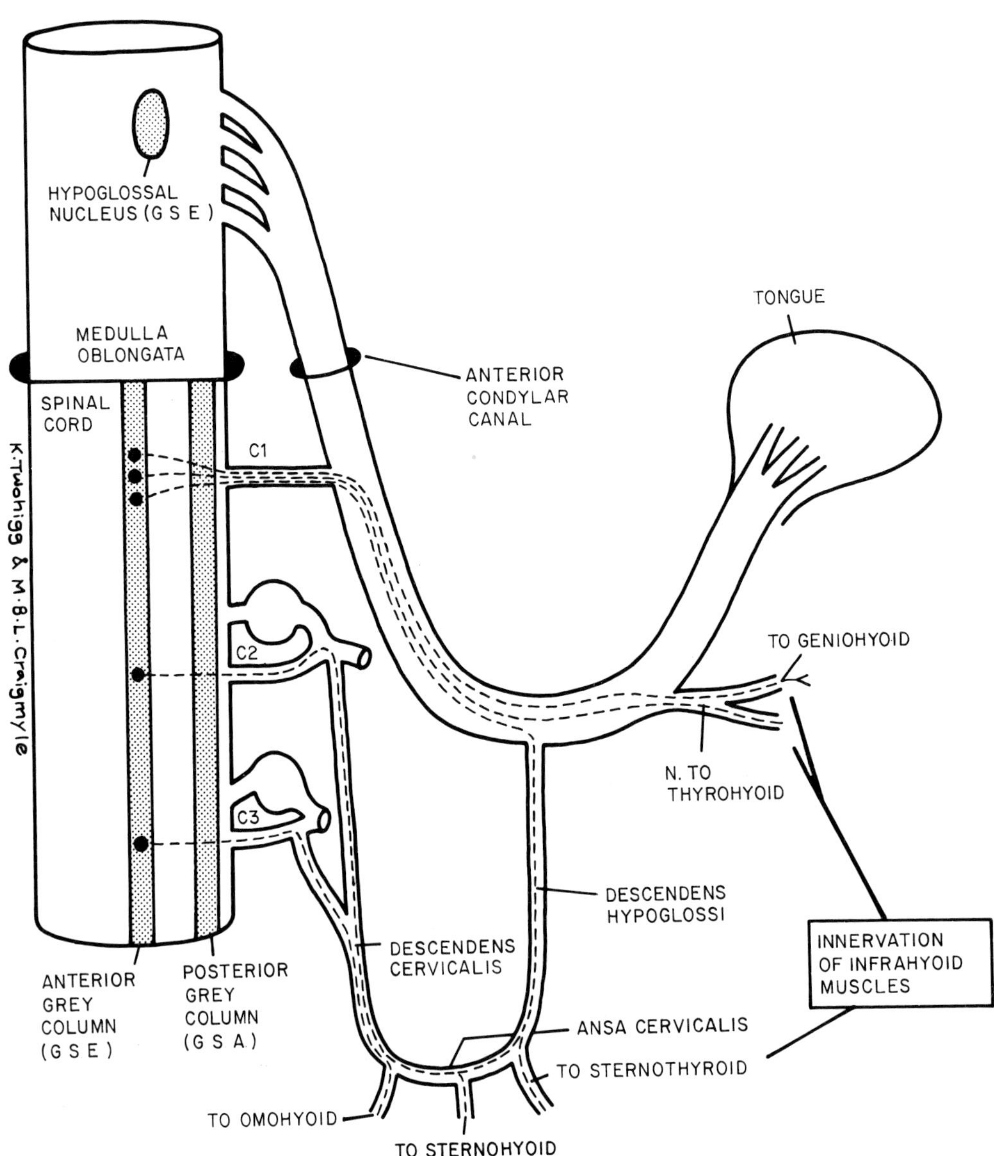

Fig 72 The distribution of the hypoglossal nerve: the spinal general somatic efferent component.

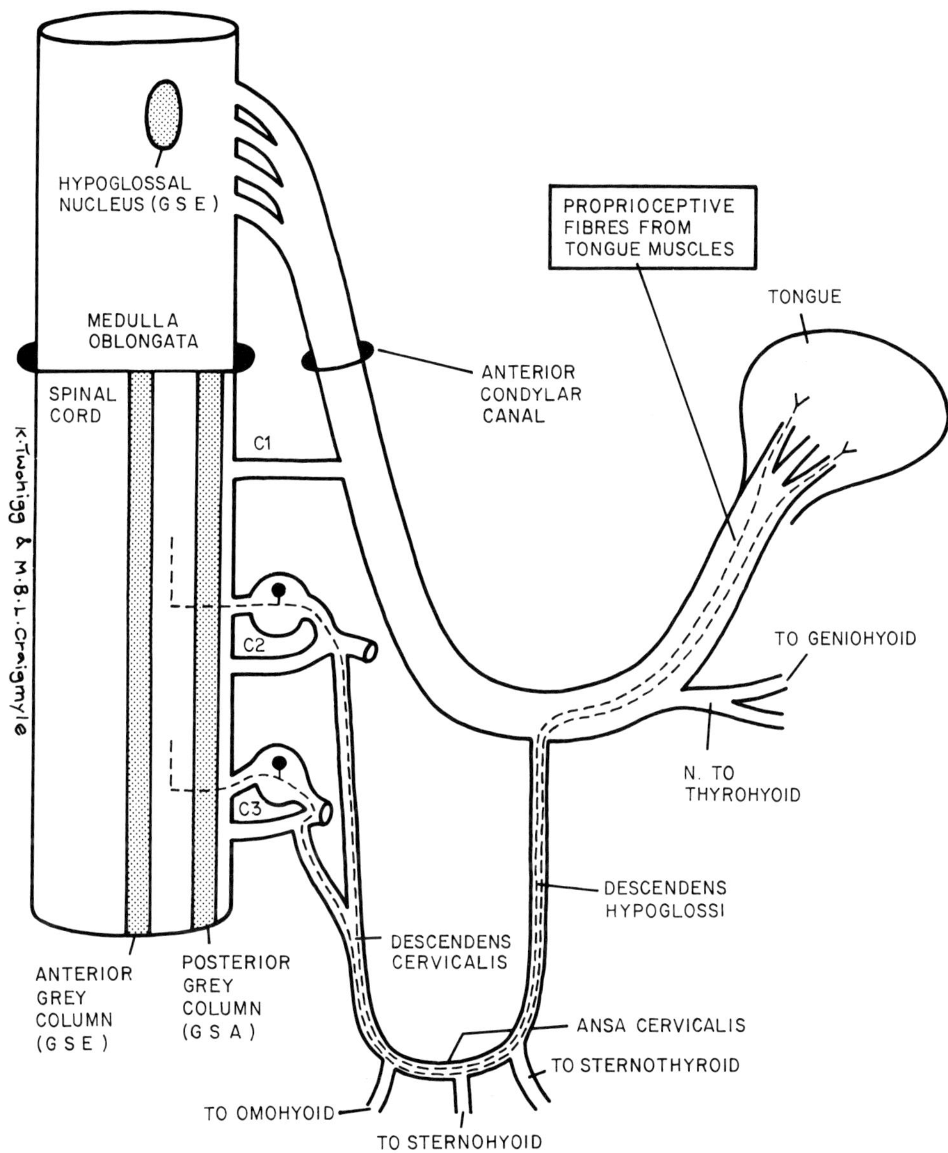

Fig 73   The distribution of the hypoglossal nerve: the general somatic afferent component.

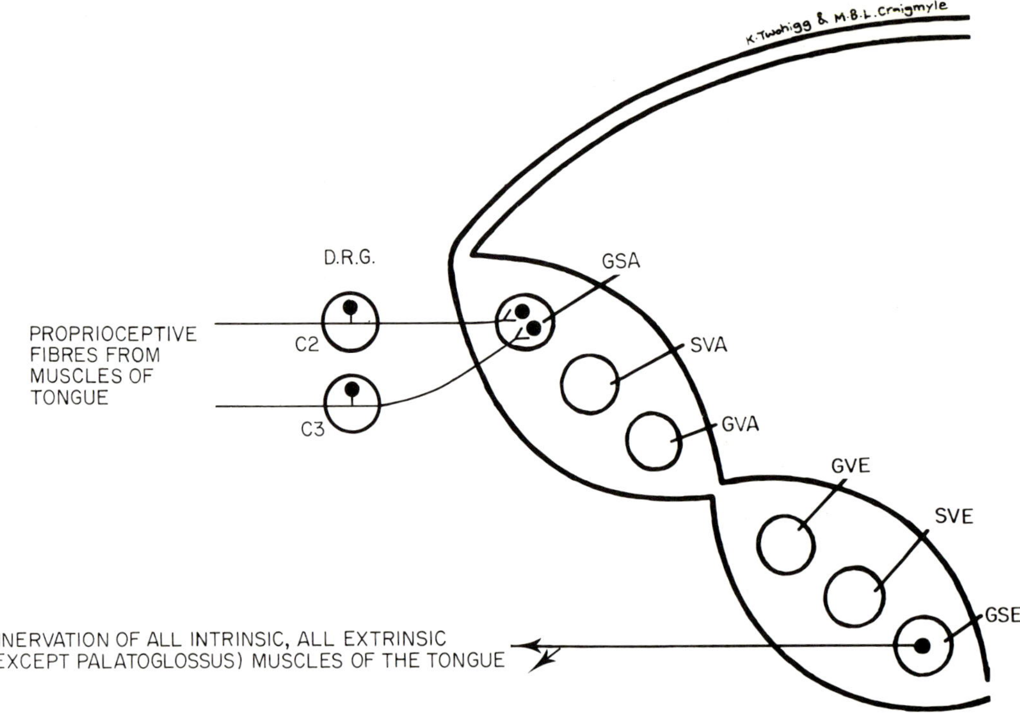

Fig 74   Summary of the nuclear connections of the hypoglossal nerve.

spinal nerves. Branches are given off from the ansa cervicalis to the sternohyoid, sternothyroid and the inferior belly of the omohyoid muscle.

The nerve to the thyrohyoid

This branch arises from the hypoglossal nerve opposite the posterior border of the hyoglossus muscle. It crosses the greater cornu of the hyoid bone to reach and supply the thyrohyoid and geniohyoid muscles.

DEEP CENTRAL CONNECTIONS OF THE HYPOGLOSSAL NERVE See Chapter 6

NUCLEAR CONNECTIONS OF THE HYPOGLOSSAL NERVE

General somatic efferent component:
1   *The hypoglossal nucleus* (Fig 71)

The axons of the lower motor neurones in the hypoglossal nucleus pass to all the intrinsic muscles of the

tongue and to all the extrinsic muscles of the tongue except palatoglossus (ie. to styloglossus, genioglossus and hyoglossus).

2   *The anterior horn of the spinal cord segments C1, C2 and C3* (Fig 72)

Fibres travel from the anterior primary ramus of C1, in the communicating branch from C1 to the hypoglossal nerve: they pass into the branch of the hypoglossal nerve to thyrohyoid muscle to supply that muscle and the geniohyoid. The C1 fibres also pass into the descending branch of the hypoglossal nerve to reach and supply the superior belly of the omohyoid muscle. Fibres from C2 and C3 pass in the anterior primary rami of these nerves into the descending cervical nerve which, as stated earlier, forms a loop (the ansa cervicalis) with the descending branch of the hypoglossal nerve. The ansa cervicalis contains, therefore, fibres from C1, C2 and C3 and supplies the sternohyoid, the sternothyroid and the inferior belly of the omohyoid muscle.

General somatic afferent component: *the dorsal root ganglia of C2 and C3* (Fig 73)

Proprioceptive fibres from the intrinsic and extrinsic muscles of the tongue are thought to be carried by the distal processes of the pseudo-unipolar nerve cells in the dorsal root ganglia of cervical spinal nerves 2 and 3: the processes pass via the hypoglossal nerve, its descending branch, the ansa cervicalis and, finally, the descending cervical nerve to reach the ganglia: the central process of the neurone enters the spinal cord and ascends in the fasciculus cuneatus to end in the cuneate nucleus. The nuclear connections of the hypoglossal nerve are summarised in Figure 74.

LESIONS OF THE HYPOGLOSSAL NERVE

A complete lesion of the nerve results in paralysis of the tongue on the affected side. With time, the affected half will atrophy. When the patient is asked to put out his tongue, it is deviated to the affected side by the unopposed action of the muscles on the unaffected side.

SITES OF LESION

See under vagus nerve. It is claimed that the nerve can become inflamed in the anterior condylar canal in a manner analagous with the involvement of the facial nerve in the facial canal.

16

POSTSCRIPT

It will be manifest, now that you have read this book, that any given mixed cranial nerve will have a minimum of two and a maximum of five nuclear connections into the six available cell columns of the brain stem. The last diagram in the book (Fig 75) provides you with six questions to ask of any mixed cranial nerve: if the answer to any question is in the affirmative, the cranial nerve concerned will be connected to one of the nuclei derived from the column in question.

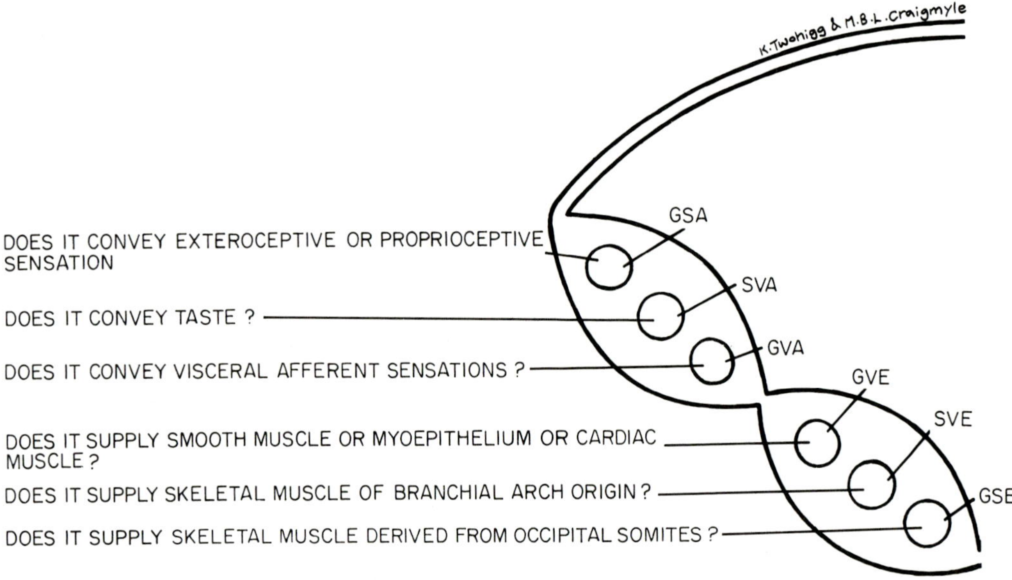

Fig 75   Six questions

INDEX

References throughout are to page numbers. If *italic*, there is a *diagram* on that page